This book is dedicated to my parents, Joan and John Huxley

Effective Community Mental Health Services

PETER HUXLEY

TERESA HAGAN

RICK HENNELLY

JENNIFER HUNT

Avebury

Aldershot · Brookfield USA · Hong Kong · Singapore · Sydney

Published by
Avebury
Gower Publishing Company Limited
Gower House
Croft Road
Aldershot
Hants GU11 3HR
England

Gower Publishing Company
Old Post Road
Brookfield
Vermont 05036
USA

British Library Cataloguing in Publication Data
Huxley, Peter
    Effective community mental health services.-(Avebury
    community care)
    1. Community mental health services
    I. Title
    362.22

    ISBN 1-85628-040-3

Printed and Bound in Great Britain by
Athenaeum Press Ltd., Newcastle upon Tyne.

Contents

Acknowledgements

We are grateful to the Department of Health for the financial support for this project, and in particular to Mary Dastgir and Pauline Williamson, who were in the Department at that time.
The research work was undertaken by Teresa Hagan with the assistance of Sara Cass.
The first drafts of the model and the chapter on accessibility were written by Teresa Hagan. The first draft of the chapters on comprehensiveness and accountability were written by Jennifer Hunt and Rick Hennely respectively. The remainder of the report was written by, and all of the subsequent editing undertaken by, the author.
We would like to thank the following people for their help and advice: Rob Langley, Manchester University Department of Psychiatry, and Janet Nicholson, and Dr. Avi Misra, Regional Computing Centre, for their hardware and software support; Esther Toye for data preparation; Dr. Jim Notman, Manchester University Department of Medicine, for expert advice on computing and data bases; Mrs. Gillian Riley, Reading Room Supervisor, the British Lending Library, Boston Spa, for her expert advice and help in locating and obtaining references; and Mrs. Pamela Rangeley, John Rylands Library, University of Manchester, for her assistance in accessing international databases.

Jacky Korer assisted in the writing of the abstracts, and she and Sylvia Edwards read and improved parts of the manuscript. Dr. Len Fagin provided enthusiastic support to the project workers, and Chris Williams assisted with the typing. Hadi Mohamad gave unstinting support to the author in the preparation of camera ready copy, and also made many amendments and corrections to the text.

The author would like to thank Professor Colin Pritchard of the University of Southampton for his detailed comments on the manuscript, and suggestions about the structure and title of the present work.

1 Development of the model used in the book

Introduction

The main aim of services for people with mental disorder is the elimination or reduction of clinical and social disablement and the achievement of an optimal quality of life for the sufferers and their carers. We agree with Wing (1988) who argues that if this is the aim of mental health policy, then it should be subject to empirical testing. Like him we feel that current policies in the UK are likely to result in mistakes in the patterns of services which are established. We exclude from this criticism the basic thrust of the Griffiths report (HMSO, 1988), but not the white paper which followed it. Most current policies are precipitous and could benefit from adjustment on the basis of findings from the research evaluations of different patterns of community service.

The overall conclusions of the present book are very much in line with these sentiments. We have arrived at our conclusions not through the taking of evidence, or site visits (although we are involved in the evaluation of a number of mental health 'centres') but on the basis of a review of empirical research into existing services. The task has required the creation of a framework within which we can consider the vast volume of writing about existing services, and their aims and outcomes. This framework is not immutable, but we have found it immensely helpful in clarifying our ideas, and in ordering the ideas of others. We find

1

the field strewn with confusions, we hope we do not add to them.

In general terms our position is that we should try to evaluate and save the best of existing practice before embarking upon wholesale and largely untested changes. This behoves us to establish what it is exactly that is useful and effective about existing services. This is not a conservative, or a reactionary position. It is not synonymous with the 'rational' position, because we recognise that service planning is only partly or indirectly affected by the evidence of research. Our position does assert that we should pay more attention to evidence than to rhetoric.

We have no doubt that the worst results occur when service planning is uninformed, or is unmotivated and uninspired, in other words when it is indifferent to the needs of mentally ill people. Mental health policy should be aiming to solve the problems of service delivery to mentally ill people, by the evaluation of what is effective, and by 'stepwise' or progressive changes in policy. Our position is in sympathy with, though again not synonymous with, an 'incrementalist' view (Booth, 1988). We hope that this book can be used by those who deliver mental health services in their struggle to provide effective services which meet the requirements of mentally ill people.

In our examination of the origins of the policy of community mental health provision in the USA we find the seeds of all the conflicting and contradictory expectations which subsequently beset the policy. We confidently expect to be able to document, in coming years similar seeds of confusion in our current mental health policy creation in the UK. In the US the original joint commission suggested that existing services should be improved, and recommended vast sums should be spent on existing services to achieve the improvement. An alternative system of community care was suggested by Anthony Celebrezze, the Director of Kennedy's cabinet level task force. He did this largely because, it seems to us, this suggestion was more in line with Kennedy's radical reforming image. It also used less money, because the financial support was only to be 'stimulatory'.

Kennedy's own goal for the policy clearly associated mental health with public health, and so in this respect was consistent with placing psychiatry within medicine, but he also sought to introduce the preventive public health model into the mental health field. Whether Kennedy realised that this model was only partly relevant to mental health seems unlikely. Kennedy, along with many others appears to be guilty of misinterpreting the writing of Gerald Caplan (Caplan,1961).

The NIMH seized the opportunity to reinterpret the policy as one for groups of people not currently in the care of psychiatric services. Professionals saw the policy as developing service which would supplement existing services. The GAO report (1974) found four other conceptions of the role of CMHCs - but we are

2

not clear where these originated. They were co-ordination of services, responsiveness to need, high quality - single standard services, and the increasing participation of state and local groups.

Not only did everyone have a view of the policy, they also had a view of what constituted a 'mental health centre' (CMHC), the cornerstone of the US policy. There is no single definition of a CMHC. Definitions of CMHCs are legion and ever changing; some hospitals were renamed CMHCs. Most CMHCs consisted of more than one service, and more than one building. In other words they were infinitely variable, as are the present services labelled CMHC in the UK. Our conclusion is that if a CMHC is a ' thing', then it is a thing like a 'cost centre' and not like a 'leisure centre'. **It is an abstract concept used to describe a network of resources based on common principles, but expressed in a variety of forms.**

The framework we have developed describes the fundamental goals of community mental health centres and community mental health services. It describes underlying principles of service delivery, in terms of ultimate aims. At the same time the elements of the model can be used as a framework for the production of operational standards of service delivery against which performance can be judged. The model is not immutable and the work of translating the research evidence into operational objectives has not been undertaken in this report. Service planners and providers are striving to offer mental health services which achieve certain fundamental goals. These goals, (and the elements of our framework) are that services should be: comprehensive; coordinated; accessible; acceptable; efficient; effective; accountable; and evaluated.

We have chosen to refer to 'Effective Community Mental Health Services' in the title of this book because we believe that effectiveness is the ultimate goal of provision. An acceptable, accessible, and well coordinated service is of little value if it is not an effective service. Evaluation (and monitoring) are crucial to the demonstration of effectiveness.

What is a community mental health centre?

There is a great deal of confusion and controversy surrounding the Community Mental Health movement in general, and CMHCs in particular. At a conference on Centres in the UK (Sayce 1987), it was suggested that the term be abandoned altogether, and that the various service initiatives using the term start calling themselves something else.

A cursory glance at such developments illustrates the problem. There are now in existence in the UK, mental health advice centres, mental health resource centres, community centres, day

3

centres, community mental health teams, in addition to those which prefer to avoid any explicit reference to mental health matters in their title (an attempt to avoid the stigmatising of clients).

It seems that those facilities calling themselves 'Centres', have little in common, and so cannot be grouped together for any useful purposes. At the most general level, it is thought that such ' Centres' are meant to be addressing the issue of prevention in psychiatry, moving away from the traditional hospital based care model, improving access to services and presumably offering something better than the services which already exist. They are regarded by some as the vanguard of change.

The type of facilities, service delivery strategies and clinical/therapeutic services which made up the CMHCs in the USA were not simply one 'thing'. In fact, this seems to be where most misunderstanding surrounding them lies, as they were not a 'thing' at all but a service delivery concept. 'Centres' were advocated as a unifying service, an umbrella facility providing the full range of services in the community (Karno & Schwartz 1974), not under one roof, or from one agency. Each centre was unique. In fact their variability, and lack of uniformity is seen as one of the problems for evaluation purposes, making their programs difficult to compare (Struening 1982).

Fiester et al (1975), notes that many of the centres in the US were hospital based. In some cases, private hospital based units became centres by ceasing to filter clients according to their ability to pay (Bolman 1972). Others were broadly based in their approach. Adler (1977), describes a centre which specialised in outreach to previously underserved groups and offered few other direct care services. Udell & Hornstra (1975), note that some centres resembled a large case work agency whose myriad of services happened to include beds and drug therapies. Some centres simply took over existing medical facilities such as free standing out patient clinics, or parts of state mental hospitals, or general hospitals (Thompson, et al 1982; Wessler, 1970; Jacobs, 1974) or medical centres wishing to expand (Lorber & Satow, 1975).

They were then " a system for the delivery of services", not as is often assumed, a building, in which services and staff were housed. 86% were the result of joining existing services (some have up to 16 member agencies) coming together in name, and these included social service agencies, out patient psychiatric clinics based in general hospitals, and many others.

Certain features have crystallised which distinguish centres from other Mental Health services, but these are neither exclusive to centres, nor necessarily definitive of them (Feldman, 1971). Given their task, which was the organising of a system of services, some requirements were laid down, and numbers of them adopted similar service delivery strategies which seemed adequate to the task. Thus they were catchmented, and required (initially) to provide the five mandatory services - inpatient services, out-patient services, emergency services, partial hospitalisation and education and consultation. Accessibility was to be a priority goal, as was continuity of care for clients, and service responsiveness.

Developments of some community services in Europe share this essential characteristic - the provision of a core set of mandated services. A number of services, for instance in eastern Europe, have a long way to go in the development of community services (Dabrowski & Stanczak, 1988). Dutch CMHCs are an amalgamation of four branches of ambulatory care - municipal social psychiatric services; private social psychiatric services; child guidance clinics and marital and family guidance centres; institutes for medical psychotherapy (which changed their name to 'multidisciplinary institutes' in the Seventies) (Schrameijer, 1987). These four have been amalgamated into Regional Institutes for Out-patient mental health (RIAGG). These are supposed to be part of the whole service coverage, and will after 1987 be funded out of hospital closure monies.

Greek CMHCs (Stefanis et al, 1985; Stefanis et al, 1986) are also an amalgamation of a range of provisions (Mavreas, 1987). These include walk-in, domiciliary and crisis intervention services; day care facilities, vocational rehabilitation; research evaluation and prevention programmes. The lesson from the literature is that it is dangerous to think of CMHCs as providing only one model of care. It is clear that no single physical location can hope to provide all the care which is required. **The 'mental health centre' describes a network of resources, based on common principles, but expressed in a variety of forms.**

UK services should strive to emulate the goals of community mental health services, but should not become tied to one service delivery strategy. The greatest danger is that the community or social service model comes to be seen as separate from the health service, or institutional model. A genuine multi-site 'centre' should include all relevant forms of service which the client and his/her family need.

US-UK Comparisons

A special conference demonstrated the growing interest in the transfer of our knowledge about mental health services across the Atlantic (Marks et al, 1988). Gittleman (1972) notes that the mental health systems in Europe and the US are similar and Feldman (1979) observes that the US problems may be different in size, but they are similar in kind. Shepherd (1987) identifies the similar problems in provision faced by the UK and US, e.g. the role of primary care in case finding, and the necessity of integrating specialist and non-specialist mental health services, in view of the fact that Mental Health specialists are unlikely to be able provide for all the need (see also Tantam 1979).

There is a growing recognition of the fact, which has been known for a long time, that mental illness is responsible for enormous social and economic costs (Frank & Kamlett, 1985). The Governments of the USA and the UK seem to have increasingly similar priorities both in terms of a market philosophy and a desire to restrict expenditure.. This trend is now being enhanced by the present UK governments' explicit investigation and adoption of US initiatives. Obvious examples include the growth in the private home based care of the elderly and the current investigations into the feasibility of adopting Health Maintenance Organisations being carried out by the Central Policy Unit. The Griffiths report, the review of the National Health Service, and the White Paper 'Caring for People', are likely to lead to the growth of private for and not-for profit organisations in the health and welfare fields in the UK. This will make our service mix more similar to that of the USA, although there will still be major differences in the way the services are funded. USA funding mechanisms seem to change with increasing rapidity and show much less stability than UK systems. However the UK funding system is becoming more heterogeneous, and although private insurance may not grow quickly, it is developing an increasingly important role.

Other similarities between the USA and the UK include plans to deinstitutionalise psychiatric care, empty mental hospitals and return patients to the community. In both countries there is a similar preoccupation with the role of 'the community', patients families (mainly women), and volunteers in the care of those with mental health problems. States in the US were instructed to set up joint planning ventures to determine the needs of each area, the resources available, and bring together all relevant agencies under the title of a centre for the delivery of coordinated care. Joint planning has been a feature of UK services for some years, although it is now under review (Hunt, 1983).

Feldman (1979) alludes to the tendency of some people to use "the banner of national differences" to obscure similarities and to block the transfer of innovations in care from one country to the other. There is no intention in the present paper to suggest that there are no differences between the two countries. The differences have been exaggerated and the number of similarities seem to be increasing from day to day, making the use of comparisons relevant and helpful.

Although Mangen (1987) feels the European states have more in common with the UK than does the US (because of their long history of state intervention) the major 'activity peaks' in social policy, around 1960, and the mid-to-late Seventies, both coincide with major developmental periods in the US. Indeed, it could be argued that the major European developments owe something to slightly earlier developments in the US. Trends in bed capacities and service utilization in the US are more like those in the UK and Italy than those in France, West Germany and Holland (Barres 1987; Haerlin, 1987; Schrameijer, 1987.)

The purpose of this book

The object of the present exercise is to review what is known about community mental health services. A particular and deliberate approach has been adopted in this book. We feel that the main considerations are the need for a conceptual clarification of the aims and objectives of CMHCs and other community based mental health services, and the need to address the pragmatic questions being asked by those who are concerned with the design of new services in the community. We are aware that contemporary service developments are taking (and will continue to take) place in an ad hoc way, often without a clear purpose, and without the benefit of empirical evidence.

It was necessary to adopt an approach which would offer some common terms of reference, encourage the identification of the similarities between the proposed changes in service provision, and offer some criteria against which they could be viewed and their performance assessed. Following Feldman's (1979) recommendations, a conceptual approach has been taken; this involved the identification of the goals of the provision, the identification of the major service delivery strategies employed, and a review of the evidence relating to their successes and failures in meeting those goals. A model was developed to organise the wealth of empirical and descriptive material on centre provision. It provides the common terms of reference necessary, draws attention to the similarities and differences in service delivery strategies, and provides a means of ordering the empirical evidence.

The model

We identified the following goals, principles and ideals in the CMHC literature. Community mental health providers (on both sides of the Atlantic) appear to strive to establish services which are: Comprehensive
      Coordinated
      Accessible
      Acceptable
      Efficient
      Effective
      Accountable
and Evaluated.

In the following sections we summarise, in a simplified form, what the literature suggests are (a) the main problems with present services and (b) the goals of future provision.

Comprehensive services

(a) At present there are limited care options available to those who need help (e.g. Blows, 1967); the type of care on offer is delivered in a way which is biased against minority groups (e.g. Littlewood & Lipsedge 1982); and the non psychiatric needs of those in care are ignored to the detriment of overall outcome (e.g. Williams & Ozarin, 1968).

(b) Services should strive to provide comprehensive coverage of an individual client's needs. At any one time, a client may need help with any or all of the following areas, psychological, social, welfare, financial, housing or health. A service should seek to offer a wider range of care options for clients. This may include increasing the volume, and scope of services to cover more client groups than are catered for at present, those underserved or overlooked by provision, or providing more services to those in greatest need.

Coordinated services

(a) At present there is a fragmented and uncoordinated referral network; finding a way around the system can baffle consumers; clients get lost between the services (e.g. Langsley 1975).

(b) A service should aim to provide a more coordinated service to its clients so that they can be referred with ease from one service to another (minimising both the risks of being overlooked and/or lost to the system). A service should competently pass information between agencies to enable a more coordinated approach to care. A coordinated service requires effective communication between the different carers involved in the care of any particular client, and the development of joint care plans. Clients requiring long term care, involving a number of different settings and carers are particularly in need of well coordinated aftercare services.

Accessible services

(a) At present many services do not reach those who may be in most need of help e.g. the poor or the most seriously ill (e.g. Fink 1979); service provision does not address the needs of certain groups e.g. the problems encountered by women, ethnic minorities (e.g. Littlewood & Lipsedge,1982); and carers. Waiting times are too long and result in poor care, or clients dropping out of treatment (e.g. Williams & Ozarin, 1968); some services are unwelcoming and offputting to those who need help (Jones,1979).

(b) The overall ideal of an accessible service is that services are accessible to all those who have mental health problems, and there are no barriers between carers and those they seek to serve. A service is thought to be more accessible if it is located near to those it seeks to serve. Long waiting times and awkward referral procedures may need to be removed and self referral extended. A service should seek to be non stigmatising. and of appreciable relevance to those in need of help. It should be in a physical setting which is pleasant, welcoming, and accessible for those with disabilities. Care should be available outside normal working hours. Clear information concerning what is available to whom and when, should be provided.

Acceptable services

(a) At present hospitals as the main site of care, are said to be overcrowded (e.g. Bratcher,1977), institutionalising (e.g. Zusman 1975; Scheper Hughes,1981), racist in practice (e.g. Littlewood& Lipsedge 1982), and stigmatising for clients (e.g. Karno & Schwartz 1974).

(b) Services should provide care options which are not damaging, which offer the least restrictive care in terms of the curtailment of liberty, and which promote self determination on the part of clients. Appropriate care should be non sexist and non racist.

Efficient services

(a) At present we do not know the most efficient combinations of forms of care; very few services are technically efficient; many are not targeted properly; and cost data used in efficiency studies are often inadequate.

(b) Services should strive to be technically efficient, and should be targeted towards priority groups. Better quality cost-effectiveness and cost utility analysis is needed. Routine monitoring should be mandatory, and common standards established.

Effective services

(a) At present we are not sufficiently knowledgeable about the most effective forms of care for different problems; our research methodologies require improvement; effective forms of long-term care have not been developed to the same level of sophistication as drug treatments for acute conditions.

(b) Services should provide the most appropriate form of care for each type of need. Effective strategies for providing for people with long-term problems should be part of the service coverage. The best combinations of different treatment elements, including professional and non professional care should be provided.

(a) At present services are dominated by professionals; citizens can often find no really useful roles in current service planning procedures; current evaluation strategies frequently exclude community representatives.

(b) Services should be accountable to a number of different 'stakeholders'; they should be democratically planned and managed with flexible and responsive mechanisms for decision making.

An attempt to document the national picture for the UK has been made by Sayce (NUPRD 1987), who carried out a postal questionnaire to all health and social service districts asking for a reporting of their current and planned initiatives in community mental heath care provision. This is the only source of data covering the picture nationally that we are aware of at the present time. Preliminary analysis of the returns appears to indicate that there are some areas where there are no planned developments. Where there are, a sizable proportion of such initiatives have adopted service delivery strategies which were prominent in the USA, for example, open door policies, multidisciplinary team working, siting centres locally and attempting some work in the broad field of preventive psychiatry.

It is clear therefore that an understanding of the impact of the concept of the community mental health centre in the US can have an important bearing on present developments in the UK. We have argued that there are good reasons why this should be the case at the present time. We hope that some of the errors of the US experience can be avoided, in particular the failure to properly evaluate a major experiment in social policy.

References

Adler, P. T. (1977 The CMHC in the Community: Another Look *Journal of Community Psychology* 5(2) p.116-123.

Barres, M. (1987) Sectorisation and overcapacity in France. *Int.J.Soc.Psychiat.* 33(2)140-143.

Blows, D (1967) Westminster Pastoral Foundation. *Counselling*, 59:20-25.

Bolman, W.H. (1972) Community Control of the C.M.H.C. *Am.J.Psychiat.*129:2.

Booth, T. (1988) *Developing Social Policy*. Gower, Aldershot.

Brandon, R.N. (1975) Differential use of mental health services In Guttentag, M. & Struening, E. *Handbook of evaluation*.

Bratcher, M. (1977) The CMHC: An Effective Approach to M.H. Care *J. of Tennessee Medical Association* 70(4):259-260

Caplan, G. (1961) *An Approach to Community Mental Health*. Tavistock, London.

Dabrowski, S. & Stanczak, T. (1988) Treatment, care and rehabilitation of the chronic mentally ill in Poland. *Hosp. Comm. Psychiat.* 39(6):657-61.

Feldman, S. (1971) Ideas and Issues in Community Mental Health. *Hosp. & Comm. Psych.* 22(11):17-21.

Feldman, S. (1979) CMHCs in the US. *J.R.Soc.Med.* 72:633-634.

Fiester, A.R., Silverman, W.H. & Beech, R.P. (1975) Problems involved in delivering emergency services in hospital based CMHCs. *J.Comm.Psychol.* 3(2):188-192.

Fink, E.B. et al (1979) Examination of clinician bias in patient referrals in partial hospitalization settings. *Hosp.Comm.Psych.*30(9):631-32.

Frank, R.G. & Kamlet, M.S. (1985) Direct costs and expenditures for mental health care in the United States in 1980. *Hosp.Comm. Psychiat.* 36:165-168.

Gittelman, M. (1972) Sectorization:The Quiet Revolution in European Mental Health Care. *Am.J.Orthopsych.* 42(1):159-167.

Griffiths, R. (1988) *Report on Community Care*. HMSO, London.

Haerlin, C. (1987) Community Care in West Germany: Concept and Reality. *Int.J.Soc.Psychiat.* 33(2):105-110.

Hunt, L.B. (1983) Community Services for Community Care. *Health Trends* 15:77-81.

Jacobs, P.E. (1974) Whither community mental health? *Int.J.M.H.* 3(2-3):35-43.

Langsley D.G. (1975) Community Mental Health: A Review of the Literature. In Barton & Sanborn, *Assessment of the CMHC Movement*.

Langsley, D.G. (1980) The CMHC: Does it treat patients? *Hosp.& Comm.Psychiat.* 31(12):816.

Littlewood, R. & Lipsedge, M. (1982) *Aliens and Alienists, Ethnic Minorities and Psychiatry*. Penguin Books.

Lorber, J. D & Satow, R. (1975) Dropout Rates in Mental Health Centres. *Social Work* 20:308-312.

Mangen, S. (1987) Mental Health Policies in Europe: An Analysis of priorities and problems. *Int.J.Soc.Psychiat*. 33(2):76-82.

Marks, I., Connolly, J. & Muijen, M. (1988) *New Directions in Mental Health Care Evaluation*. Institute of Psychiatry, London.

Mavreas, V.G. (1987) Greece:The Transition to Community Care. *Int.J.Soc.Psychiat*. 33(2):154-164.

Sayce, L. (1987) *CMHCs Conference Report*. National Unit for Psychiatric Research & Development, London.

Scheper-hughes, N. (1981) Dilemmas in deinstitutionalisation. *J.Operational Psychol*. 12(2):90-99.

Schrameijer, F. (1987) New Comprehensive Mental Health Authorties in the Netherlands. *Int.J.Soc.Psychiat*. 33(2): 132-136.

Shepherd, M. (1987) Mental Illness and primary care. *Am.J.Pub.Health*:12-13.

Stefanis, C., Kounalaki, A., Madianos, M. & Madianou, D. (1985) *The first Community Mental Health Centre in Greece: Three years assessment of an experiment*. Plenum Press, New York.

Stefanis, C., Madianos, M.G. & Gittelman, M. (1986) Recent developments in the care, treatment, and rehabilitation of the chronic mentally ill in Greece. *Hosp. Comm. Psychiat*. 37(10):1041-1044.

Struening, E.L. (1982) Evaluation in CMHC program: A Bold New Approach. In Neigher, *Evaluation and Program Planning*.

Tantam, D. & Burns, B.J. (1979) An international comparison of two systems of community mental health care. *Psych.Med*. 9:541-550.

Thompson, J.W. et al (1982) Past- now 50 years of psychiatric services 1940-1990. *Hosp. & Comm. Psychiat*. 33:711-717.

Udell, B. & Hornstra, R.K. (1975) Good patients and Bad. *Arch.Gen.Psychiat*. 32:1533-37.

Wessler, R.L. et al (1970) Social characteristics of patients readmitted to a CMHC. *Comm.M.H.Journal* 6(1):69.

Williams,R.H. & Ozarin, L. (1968) *Community Mental Health*. Jossey Bass, New York.

Wing, J.K. (1988) *Mental health policy in the UK*. Royal Society Lecture, London.

Zusman, J. (1975) Philosophic basis for a community and social psychiatry. In Barton & Sanborn. *op cit*.

2 Comprehensive and coordinated services

Introduction

> Coordination is '... the most sought after, but the most elusive, operational component in comprehensive mental health care systems in all countries' (WHO 1977).

The ideal of providing a comprehensive and coordinated service to the individual in receipt of care is widely accepted as a major goal of all mental health care programmes. The Royal College of Psychiatrists (1987) has included these service aspects in their recent joint statement with carers, as elements of good mental health service' and the DHSS (1975) have also stressed that 'the hallmark of a good service for the mentally ill is a high degree of local coordination'.

The most overt attempt to provide a comprehensive and coordinated services to a specific population was the development of CMHCs in the USA. The provision of an integrated range of services was one of the central ideas underpinning the programme (Feldman 1979). Coordination and comprehensiveness were two of the nine goals examined by Dowell & Ciarlo (1983).

Continuity of care and the coordination of services is vitally important in the U.K at the present time as services undergo change and diversification. Freeman (1976) has pointed out that we are moving from a situation of all-embracing care previously provided by the mental hospital, to a 'dispersed institution' which has the objective of 'providing a continuous spectrum of services (medical and social) as a comprehensive arrangement, for a defined population'. Foley & Sharfstein (1983) defined the task at hand as that of converting the chaotic 'de facto mental health system into an intentional system of rationalised care'.

The reasons for wanting to provide comprehensive and coordinated services are not simply 'clinical-humanitarian' (i.e. important for patient outcome) but also, as Schulberg & Bromet (1981) point out, 'fiscal-political'. Any service which is not coordinated can hardly claim to be efficient and effective (see chapter on effectiveness). The skills of staff, however good, will be wasted if they do not consult and cooperate in their support of individuals and families (Bennet 1978). Additional resources and more services may be needed, but there is widespread support for the view that the efficiency of current provision can be improved by increasing the coordination of existing services (Test 1981; Sayce,1987). Aiken (1988) suggests that successful community services require the following characteristics: a comprehensive range of settings and services, with varying levels of supervision, that provides realistic alternatives to institutional care; assignment of clearly defined and continuing responsibility for each chronically mentally ill person in the community; and budgetary control over the broad range of relevant services and settings, with fiscal incentives for providing appropriate and cost-effective care.

The success of providing comprehensive and coordinated services by the use of different organisational and administrative strategies has rarely been systematically assessed. The research which relates to problems of integration and comprehensive provision in mental health services is examined in this chapter.

The concepts of 'comprehensive' and 'coordinated'

Very few attempts have been made to clarify the characteristics that comprehensive and coordinated services should embrace and how these should be systematically operationalised. It would appear that there are, as yet, no clearly articulated standards by which different services and programmes can be compared (Zusman 1972). Hodges (1970) stressed the importance of avoiding unrealistic expectations of the performance of community mental health services in terms of comprehensive and coordinated provision.

Inconsistent use of the terms 'comprehensive' and 'coordinated', both in general and in relation to different aspects of service provision, has probably contributed to the confusion in this area. Coordination has been seen as subsumed in the definition of a comprehensive service (Belleck & Mueser 1986) or as encompassing comprehensiveness as one of it's own features (Bachrach

1981). Clearly, the two concepts are not entirely independent, but the distinctions between them need to be clarified to promote comparability of studies and identification of further research needs.

Exactly what is to be coordinated and whose needs are to be met comprehensively are rarely articulated. Small mental health initiatives are often judged inadequate because they are not providing a 'comprehensive service', when they are actually aimed at complementing existing services, or providing comprehensive care for one specific target group or geographical area.

Comprehensive **coverage of the mental health needs of a population** is the first meaning of this term. Comprehensive coverage can mean the inclusion of all the relevant general and specialist psychiatric services, that is, all general and liaison psychiatry, forensic psychiatry, child psychiatry, the psychiatry of old age, substance abuse, etc. (This is the way the Royal College of Psychiatrists tends to see it). It can also mean the inclusion of all treated and untreated disorder, that is, conspicuous and hidden morbidity, as well as efforts to prevent disorder from occurring in high risk populations.

The second meaning of the term is the comprehensive **provision of services**. This is a problematic idea, because it is hard to say what constitutes the total possible range of services which might be provided. When comprehensive service provision is described in the American literature it includes the five mandated services of the CMHC legislation i.e out patient care, in patient care, partial hospitalisation, emergency services, and consultation and education. This excludes the non-psychiatric and voluntary sector services which might be needed. This conception of 'comprehensive service' is a very specific one, and is perhaps the one which is most prevalent in the US literature. However very similar descriptions of the elements which make up a comprehensive service can be found in most European countries. As we have already seen a group or network of related services, rather than a community based 'resource centre' building, was the original meaning of the term CMHC in the US.

Comprehensive **care of the individual client's needs** is the third way in which the term is used. The achievement of comprehensive care for the individual service user, depends both on the structural aspects of the availability of the different care options, and the coordination of those to best meet the various needs of the client. In this sense the comprehensive service should not neglect medical needs (physical or psychiatric) by concentrating only on psychosocial needs, or vice versa. A comprehensive service should not neglect what Bachrach (1980) has called the 'central functions' of a service for those with long term problems - treatment, custody, and asylum.

Thus the comprehensiveness and the coordination of services can be examined either in relation to the needs of the particular client or target population which is the concern of the service, or in relation to the needs of the particular catchment population within which services are located. These two perspectives may lead to the examination of different issues and the suggestion of different service strategies. The services available to an area can be studied in terms of the different client groups' views of services, or from a service perspective e.g how does the known need for services relate to the local pattern of provision.

In the following sections comprehensive and coordinated coverage of the needs of the individual client has been examined separately from the provision of comprehensive and coordinated mental health services to the whole range of mental health problems in any population. In each section the research methods will be reviewed. Subsequently, the research which relates to the various attempts to increase coordination and range of mental health service provision will be discussed.

The coordination of care for the individual

The coordination of individual care is most often defined in service terms as the 'rapid movement of patients between services as their needs dictate'(Feldman 1971). Continuity is similarly defined as 'the relatedness between past and present care in conformity with the therapeutic needs of the client' (Bass & Windle 1972). Needs are usually defined by service providers.

Bass & Windle (1972) provide a method for measuring continuity of patient care as it relates to the needs of the patient as they are perceived by the therapist. In their study the appropriate resources were available at the centre under scrutiny or at other agencies 99% of the time, but in 38% of the sample continuity was not maintained because clients/families rejected treatment, missed appointments or sought help elsewhere. Bass & Windle's method could be used for comparing services along the continuity of care dimension as perceived by therapists.

Their operational categories were; client movement or lack of it with respect to need, stability of client-caretaker relationships, written/verbal communication concerning clients, and efforts made to retrieve those dropping out of treatment. They judged that much of the information required to maintain continuity of care was available in client records.

Hagedorn (1976) has described how 'Management Information Systems' (or computerised case registers) (see also evaluation chapter) can be designed to monitor and evaluate client utilisation of various services and client movement between different elements of the service. This approach can tell us about the variety and quantity of care received by an individual but misses out the essential element of the appropriateness of providing him/her with these forms of care, and is measuring merely service rather than individual outcomes. As Dowell & Ciarlo (1983) point out, the most common barrier to continuity of care is client drop out rather than service problems. This may illustrate one of hazards of overlooking the client perspective on the appropriateness of services. Cline and Sinnott (1981) have suggested the use of comparative case study methods to examine the effect of organisational change on clients.

Staff time utilisation studies have also been used to investigate the coordination of care for the individual client (Harakal 1975), these will be discussed more fully when the research relating to team working is reviewed.

Comprehensive care for the individual

It is widely accepted that those seeking help within the mental health delivery system will have multiple 'bio-psycho-social' needs, which may need the appropriate skills and intervention of more than one agency (DHSS 1983). Many of these agencies may not be recognised as specifically providing mental health services. Comprehensive programs have been described, particularly for long-term patients (Belleck & Mueser 1986; Antinnen 1985; Lamb 1980; Test & Stein 1978). All of these programs emphasise the importance of such things as housing and accommodation, employment and occupation, education, caring for carers, advice, social and leisure activities, income support, transport and other practical help as well as a range of specific interventions, together with the provision of general health care (Royal College of Psychiatrists 1987). In theory, in most programs, these services are tailored into a package according to the person's needs.

Belleck & Mueser (1986) have suggested that the variety of services offered to a client will be more important than the amount of individual therapy which they receive. Grad (1968) has emphasised the importance of providing support to those caring for clients. The inclusion of services for carers has assumed considerable significance over the last twenty years. Following the publication of 'Schizophrenia at Home' (Creer & Wing,1974) the size and contribution of the National Schizophrenia Fellowship, and the North West Fellowship has grown.

A comprehensive and coordinated service for a population

The success of a service in providing care for all those in need of help in a catchment area can be studied by comparing service utilisation and needs assessment data (see efficiency chapter). This may be facilitated by the specific targeting of a particular group or mental health problem by parts of the service so that coverage is comprehensive, in the sense that it meets the needs of that particular group of clients.

There have been a number of studies looking into the interrelations of various agencies in their efforts to provide a comprehensive mental health service. It has been noted however that such studies are 'more interesting for the range of strategies suggested than for quantitative data' (NORC 1971). Dowell and Ciarlo (1983) did not cite any studies of inter-agency coordination in their review of the CMHCs programme.

NORC (1971) conducted their own study of the relationship of nine CMHCs with other caregiving agencies in terms of the proportion of staff time spent in consultation and education, and the number of referrals to and from the different agencies. The staff in the CMHCs and the other helping agencies had a poor understanding of the concept of coordinated care. Unfortunately the questionnaires used in this study did not define the concepts involved, and were restricted to the subjective views of the staff concerning the centre's success in providing a more coordinated service. One staff member in a New Orleans' CMHC gave a graphic view of the coordination of care in that city when she said 'Nothing in New Orleans is really organised, except vice'.

Components of a comprehensive service system

When a comprehensive service is described in the American literature it nearly always comprises a listing of the 'five mandated services' i.e out patient care, in patient care, partial hospitalisation, emergency services, and consultation and education. This was increased to twelve in 1975, and then included specialist services to elderly people and those with drug and alcohol problems. Each centre had to provide these services. The situation in this country is very different, as many areas already provide many of these services to the populations they serve. The new 'rash' of Community Mental Health Centres in the UK is more likely to be 'filling gaps' in the current services, for example caring for one particular group or underserved population, than taking on all these functions.

A review of current criticisms

Conspicuous morbidity

As has already been noted, there is widespread agreement that services tend to have uncoordinated and fragmented referral systems that clients may be 'lost' in the system, or not picked up by the services sufficiently quickly (Langsley 1975).

Blows (1967) criticises the limited nature of care options available to those seeking help, and it is generally accepted that certain groups of clients are more likely to receive inappropriate forms of care, for example black people (Littlewood 1986), or that those in need of help may find themselves inappropriately in the criminal system (Eysenck,1987; Stelovich, 1979). The high utilisation rates of emergency services at general hospitals, particularly by known clients (Blaney & West 1987, Haw 1987) is another indication that the psychiatric services are often not able to deal with all the needs of all their clients.

There are several articles which examine the problems caused by concentrating exclusively on certain aspects of treatment whilst neglecting the range of non-psychiatric needs of those seeking help, and that this is generally to the detriment of overall outcome (Williams 1968). It is important to note that most of the criticisms of the comprehensiveness and coordination of services to clients has been documented by studies which have included the client's perspective.

Burgoyne et al (1979) conducted a study at an out-patient clinic which monitored patients' requests to staff. Staff significantly underestimated the importance that patients attach to their requests and there was a disparity between patients' and therapists' perceptions of important needs.

Yamanoto (1984) found that systematically orienting therapists to a client's culture, expectations and needs before therapy led to increased client satisfaction and coping. Clients were more likely to feel that their needs had been met appropriately than clients seeing therapists who had not been 'oriented' in this way. The effects seen were independent of the therapists' experience, clients' ethnicity and their orientation towards psychotherapy. It would be useful to know whether 'drop out' rates are reduced by such interventions, and thus whether continuity of care is facilitated. Murray (1975) similarly emphasised the importance of concentrating on the culture and community of those seeking help from community mental health centres.

The role of families and supporters in influencing 'outcome' has sometimes been overlooked in psychiatric service evaluations. Gilleard (1987) sampled consecutive referrals for psychiatric day care and found that poor outcome in terms of subsequent institutionalisation was influenced when emotional distress was initially reported in supporters and was not alleviated. Hunt (1983) suggests that the statutory services should support relatives and neighbours upon whom the success of independent living so often depends.

Ebringer and Christie-Brown (1980) examined two samples of newly admitted short-stay psychiatric patients and found that nearly 30% of people changed address whilst in hospital or were discharged without known accommodation. A one day sample of people in the day hospital and wards showed that 28.4% came from transitory accommodation or had no fixed abode, 64.7%

were unemployed and 50% living alone. Of the in patients 40.5 % were homeless and 36.5% had no visitors. The authors suggest that many patients have lost their community supports by the time they reach hospital.

Birch (1983) documented, by means of case histories, the difficulties which people who had suffered from mental illness experienced in the field of employment and occupation. She also noted that for some, problems of housing and loneliness were just as pressing but that little help was available to relieve these problems.

All of these studies highlight the need to see clients in relation to the context in which they live, and to address the compliment of needs which they present to mental health services. Dowell & Ciarlo (1983), in their review of CMHC services concluded that although the range of services available to clients was greater than before, there had not been much success at increasing the coordination of services, mainly it seemed because of what they call 'resistant drop outs', who may make up as much as 40% of clientele, who thwart coordination efforts. Studies identifying the reasons for this high proportion of people leaving services are needed.

Clients with long term problems

The most widely documented criticisms of the coordination and range of care available for those involved with the psychiatric services relates to the fate of long term sufferers. Schwartz et al (1983) suggest that the care of this group is characterised by the fragmented relationship between providers, the fragmented authority between systems and fragmented goals and objectives in general. It was suggested that this fragmentation was an inevitable consequence of a system with multiple agencies and professions who have different goals and values.

People are often discharged to inadequate or non-existent facilities (Feldman 1979, Reich 1973a, 1973b) or remain, inappropriately, in mental hospitals (Specht 1983) because of accommodation problems. Others have documented in more detail the fates of those discharged from hospital (see also the effectiveness of aftercare, effectiveness chapter). For example, Johnstone et al (1984) followed up 120 patients with diagnoses of schizophrenia discharged from a hospital over a five year period. 66 were out of hospital and willing to be interviewed. More than 50% were judged to have 'psychotic' features, and although no interviewees sought readmission to hospital many had severe emotional, social and financial problems. 27% had no contact with any medical or social services. The authors also documented the unmet needs of the relatives involved and the fact that frequent changes in staff for those in contact with the services lead to poor continuity of services. Many informants and relatives would have preferred a system where one person remained in charge of their case and was aware of all the relevant details. The authors conclude that the services were severely limited in dealing with the chronicity and severity of the impairments resulting from schizophrenic illness.

Bachrach (1982) examines the research concerning community support systems for chronic patients and emphasises the discrimination against this group which exists in the present system of care (Presidents Commission 1978) which is geared towards those with motivation and insight. Advocacy for those with lack of volition was cited as a basic requirement, since even when they are the target of a specific programme the breadth of their needs is seriously underestimated.

Bachrach (1982) quotes Gruber et al (1978) who call for programmes which provide a "response to the real but unarticulated needs that are not being met by the mental health system". Studies incorporating the perspectives of clients will be more useful in highlighting the problems of services in respect of comprehensiveness and coordination. Service oriented studies may be useful in examining the effects of policy changes on service outcomes such as drop out rates and interagency interactions.

Hoult (1986) and others (Test & Stein 1980, Fenton et al 1979) stress that 'good' outcome depends essentially on providing programmes which are comprehensive and continuous in respect of individual care. Important ingredients would be intensive initial help, active involvement of the patient and the family in planning, consistent care by one team, a personal case manager, assertive but not intrusive intervention, practical help, a 24 hour service with rapid response and an on-going extensive service.

Hunt (1983) points to the problems of planning comprehensive programmes between health, social services and voluntary agencies, caused by their different structures and different understanding of the problems involved. The problems to be overcome are illustrated by a director of social services: 'If you wanted to create a structure for health and social services that inhibited cooperation and lead to misunderstanding and inertia, you could do no better than reinvent the present structure'.(Social Services Select Committee, 1984)

The complex problems facing long term sufferers will require a multi-agency and 'multifaceted' approach to community support systems (Keith 1978) which is able to cater for housing needs, financial problems,and provide support to families and carers. Coordination will have to be actively pursued by providers (Test 1981) because, while clients and families understand the complexity of the services which face them, they are not always able to engage successfully with them, and have only a marginal influence on the shape, performance, and relationships between the elements of the total service system. Their influence is reduced by the fact that so many different services are required to meet their needs. The increasing complexity of services has increased the justification for the existence of a 'case manager' who can be accountable to the client for arranging and coordinating the care provided by a multitude of agencies.

Schulberg & Bromet (1981) point out that most studies lean (dramatically) towards the rhetorical and away from the empirical. We have tried to confine our examination of the effectiveness of services to the latter type of paper. We have found, particularly in relation to the evaluation of services, that most papers display the unfortunate tendency identified by Schulberg & Bromet (see also the chapter on evaluation).

Hidden morbidity and high risk groups

In addition to their failure to adequately or coherently meet the needs of those formally recognised as requiring some form of service, current specialist psychiatric services only deal with a small proportion of the 'pool' of morbidity that exists in the community. The lack of attention to morbidity which, in many cases, might be preventable by timely intervention is another issue raised by the critics of current patterns of service provision. The barriers to the identification and successful treatment of morbidity in its early stages are many and complex (see Broskowski & Baker 1974; and the effectiveness chapter); and yet there are known associations between various forms of stress, for example unemployment, and mental health problems (Pritchard, 1988).

There have been a number of studies examining psychiatric morbidity in primary care attenders (for a review of this work, see Goldberg & Huxley, 1980). For example Goldberg (1976) found primary care attenders to be more psychiatrically disturbed than a random sample of the local population. Kessler et al (1977) found 21.7% prevalence of psychiatric morbidity in medical service users as compared to 16.7% in non-users. Women tended to present with affective disorders and males with substance abuse problems. The authors stressed the need to train G.P.s to recognise and refer psychiatric problems to the appropriate services.

Skuse & Williams (1984) found a prevalence of 34% psychiatric disorder in general practices and recommended screening to aid recognition of those in need of help. Regier et al (1978) estimated that 60% of all patients in the United States with emotional disorders are seen and supported in the primary care system. Because of the evidence of a lack of collaboration, there has a been a widespread call for the integration of mental health and primary health care services. The research relating to this issue will be reviewed below.

Aspects of unmet and preventable need in the community, and

how mental health services have addressed the problems will be more fully examined in the chapter on 'accessibility' in this volume.

Attempts to improve coordination and comprehensiveness

Introduction

In order for services to become more coordinated and comprehensive in their provision, for both the individual seeking care and the mental health needs of their catchment area, various 'service features' and systems have been adopted. Many of these have become characteristically associated with the community mental health centre movement, but can also be found as new features of traditional services and small scale community projects. Some features are 'added on' to services to co-ordinate an individual's care, others involve some reorganisation of services to increase the coordination between them.

Perhaps because of the documented methodological difficulties in this area of enquiry (Cowen 1978), there is a shortage of research which examines the effectiveness of these attempts to improve coordination and comprehensiveness. Leaf (1985) also notes a lack of research on the effects of institutional environments on the distribution, nature and volume of service provided.

Each of the following sections does not address the issue of the effectiveness or efficiency of the service features discussed (which is covered elsewhere) but relates specifically to the literature concerning the provision and amelioration of services in respect of their integration and the range of care they offer.

Multidisciplinary teams

If the separate disciplines are poorly coordinated because of geographical, organisational, and accessibility problems, as is so often suggested, then an obvious solution would be to place them all under one roof, with common service goals and referral systems. The solution is not so simple, as a large number of papers confirm.

Bloom (1976) surveyed staff members and program directors about interdisciplinary functioning and training in their centres. He found that this way of working was the rule rather than the exception. The author lists some of the advantages of this approach, and suggest that ultimately co-operative activity 'enhance organisational effectiveness in general and service delivery to patients in particular'. He also suggests that the outcome of a well functioning team effort can be significantly greater than the cumulative effects of the discrete performance of the individual practitioners. There is little indication in the current literature as to whether this is true in practice, or which models of team functioning would lead to better performance.

Bloom's survey showed highly significant differences by profession in the proportion of 'interdisciplinary interactions' reported. For example psychiatrists report that they spend 81.5% of their time in 'interdisciplinary interactions' and mental health workers 44.9%, of their time. Most workers agreed that a formal procedure existed for team meetings (85%) and that contributions to team discussions were judged on merit rather than discipline (85%). 75% believed that the interdisciplinary approach was superior when it came to interagency collaboration and coordination and working with community groups etc. Nurses and 'other' personnel expressed the greatest preference for interdisciplinary working, psychiatrists and psychologists expressed the least preference.

Replies solicited on an 'Egalitarian Functioning Scale' showed that psychiatrists scored substantially lower than all other groups. It seems that practitioners, particularly psychiatrists, often agree with the interdisciplinary approach while retaining a hierarchical attitude to task assignment. In the light of these discrepancies Bloom (1976) suggests a more detailed analysis of team functioning and the modes and consequences of interdisciplinary training. Bloom's findings were repeated in a study of multidisciplinary ward rounds in a district general hospital psychiatric unit in the UK (Sanson-Fisher et al,1979).

Feldman (1978) has stressed the importance of training. He suggests that, on the whole, the education of mental health professionals does not equip them for work in community mental health centres, and that training should ideally be 'unidisciplined', relating wholly to the needs of patients and free from the inherent constraints of traditional models, which will perpetuate the 'overpromise and under performance' cycle of mental health programmes.

In both Bloom's study (1976) and an earlier study by Glasscote (1969) staff reported training needs in the areas of consultation and prevention as well as the improvement of clinical skills, particularly in family and group therapy.

Staff time utilisation studies may give some useful clues to the nature and extent of interdisciplinary working in mental health programmes. One study compares different facilities on this dimension (Seigel et al 1983). A two week observation of 193 staff was conducted in 18 different facilities. They found major differences in the amount of direct patient contact between private and state funded facilities, the former staff spending twice as much time in this activity. State funded staff spent more time in record-use activities (usually relating to quality assurance!) and staff-patient ratios were lower. For psychiatrists, psychologists and social workers the largest single activity was interstaff communication. Psychiatrists spent 23% of their time on 'personal activities'. In out patient facilities about 40% of time was spent in direct client contact. The authors suggest that a high proportion of time is spent in communication with other professionals because of the existence of multidisciplinary teams!

Harakal (1975) developed an instrument to assess staff time utilisation in a CMHC, which they suggested could be used to compare disciplines and clinics and to evaluate the impact of policy changes. They documented improvements in clinical and financial efficiency after introducing the 'logging' to their centre. Lang (1982) set out to study whether a community mental health team approach lead to more democratic working relationships and more socially oriented 'holistic' treatment of clients, which are two of the main goals often cited for this working method. She found no questioning of competence in case assignment meetings and staff relationships appeared initially non-deferential. However, closer observation showed that nurses were doing all the 'bothersome' expediting work such as contacting people who missed appointments and that in addition psychiatry students were offered the 'good' clients as an inducement to work with the centre. Lang observed that labour was still divided along traditional hierarchical lines, although these differences were initially concealed by a 'zeal for a democratic culture', there was in reality little or no discussion of cases by the team, before or after assignment.

Another group of papers relates more specifically to the problems that psychiatrists experience working in community mental health settings. As a profession they appear to have had the most difficulties with this way of working. Leong (1982) suggests that 'good' psychiatrists have no choice but to leave CMHCs because CMHCs espouse a social service model of care. He also suggests that ideally psychiatrists should be the team leaders to ensure that patient's biomedical needs are met. Donovan (1982) also point to many problems perceived by psychiatrists in CMHCs and suggest that these could be alleviated if centres were allied to university departments of psychiatry, and community psychiatrists were given more support.

Fink and Weinstein (1979) suggest that the increasing dissatisfaction with psychiatrists in CMHCs was due to conflicts over authority and control. Reinstein (1978) surveyed psychiatrists working in CMHCs and found that many were unhappy with the continuity of care and also with their relegation to signing prescriptions and accountability to non-medical administrators and directors. They also disliked having to treat "all patients" and the authors suggest that private practice is more appropriate to psychiatrists needs since "there is more respect for the doctor-patient relationship".

It is clear that despite the promise which a well-functioning team could hold, there may be a need to address more fundamental issues concerning the barriers to interdisciplinary interaction, before the ideal is realised. The issues involved have been well documented , in relation to doctors and social workers by Huntingdon (1981). It is clear that merely forming workers from different agencies and backgrounds in to a 'team' is no guarantee of increasing the coordination and cooperation between them. In some cases it is even possible that the reverse could occur, and that it may also do little to promote interagency cooperation, especially when workers in other agencies are not working as teams.

There seems to be a dearth of research relating specifically to the question of whether clients referred to a interdisciplinary team setting actually receive more coordinated care or whether teams are able to meet a wider range of the needs of the clients and groups that they serve. More research is needed to identify the team and organisational structures which tend to produce better outcomes, as well as into the reasons for the failure of some teams to function adequately from their own and the client's point of view. The optimal mix of input from professional and nonprofessional sources will have to be identified for a wide range of different client circumstances.

Key workers

The key worker concept is the second service feature which is often proposed as a method of increasing the coordination and range of care provided to the individual client. Again there seems to be little practice based research into its real advantages. Although, as we have already suggested, clients may prefer this system, the subject has not been systematically investigated. Multidisciplinary teams often feature a key worker system (Lang 1982).

The professionals who are the subject of most papers are community psychiatric nurses, closely followed by social workers. Most papers are anecdotal or descriptive (for example, Albini, 1963; Maisey, 1975; Henderson, 1973 a,b,c; Lancaster, 1980; Whitehead, 1987; and Hunter, 1980). Griffith and Mangen (1980) reviewed the literature relating to CPNs and concluded that there has been sparse evaluation of the respective roles, and liaison between, CPNs, psychiatrists , G.Ps and social workers, but 'nonetheless the articles give a clear indication that CPNs play an invaluable role in the community through a worthwhile and effective service' both as part of MDTs as well as sole professionals. They suggest that the overlapping roles of professionals should be examined to eliminate conflict and duplication. Wooff (1986) however found that there was little evidence of the efficiency of community psychiatric nurses, and, in her sample, a comparison group of psychiatric social workers were better able to plan their work, to select appropriate targets for intervention, and to use other services on behalf of clients.

In sum, we are still short of evidence to the effect that clients with key workers receive care with a higher level of continuity than those in the 'traditional' system and whether they are offered a wider range of care or care with a better outcome. The functioning of the keyworker under different organisational structures should also be the subject of research, for example, as part of a MDT, attached to the hospital or the G.P. It is likely that the method of working and interdisciplinary liaison will vary in each case. The client perspective of key worker services is also lacking (Hoshall and Friedman 1975).

Joint planning

Joint planning is recommended in the search for comprehensive, coordinated, cost-effective, non-duplicative mental health care (e.g Hunt 1983). There seems to be no research which directly relates to our current concern of comparing the functioning of different schemes along these dimensions. Wistow (1987) reports that a survey in the UK found that the impact of joint funding on collaboration between health and social services was limited, compared to the level of collaboration that was hoped for from the policy. It is important to bear in mind that efforts to stimulate joint initiatives in the community have not been funded at anything like the level necessary to provide a genuine incentive to alter the balance of services away from hospital care.

Sharfstein (1978) and Pepper & Ryglewicz (1982) have stressed that funding patterns may present barriers to effective service coordination; how can one service actively co-ordinate another if they are funded by different sources? This is an important consideration in the U.K. The Audit Commission (1986) have pointed to the funding problems of local authorities, who, in attempting to provide mental health services are 'penalized through the rate support system for building the very community services which government favours.' The problem of funding community services from hospital closures serves to exacerbate the tensions between areas of service which should be regarded as complementary rather than in competition. This tendency has been observed in Dutch services (Schrameijer, 1987).

Putting social policies into action is a complex business, and joint planning seems to combine the individual and shared problems of the organisations which may be reluctantly brought together to construct and implement policy. Joint planning can be handicapped by the organisations' different short term preoccupations, the failure to achieve a common philosophy and principles, the absence of compatible information systems (or the presence of conflicting ones), the different accountability systems and priorities of the parent bodies. Some advocates of the joint approach seem to be unperturbed by the problems which follow from situations of 'dual influence', where individual workers are the subject of two different lines of accountability (e.g Towell & McAusland, 1984).

Consultation and education

Preventive consultation and educational work has been adopted by community mental health services to encourage comprehensive coverage of the mental health needs of the populations they serve. (See the chapter on effectiveness for a consideration of the outcome of this effort.)

NORC (1971) studied liaisons between several CMHCs and local agencies such as the police. They found some impact on the coordination of services but no effect on the comprehensiveness of services provided. Adler (1977) describes the role of a C & E service in finding service gaps for those traditionally receiving no help, he emphasises the importance of seeing such activities as on a continuum with clinical services.

In a survey of thirty community mental health centres, Nuehring (1979) produces an analysis which suggests that the preventive activity and emphasis of a centre will depend largely on the type of interactions which it has with other agencies; negotiations, cooptations or coalitions. He gives no analysis of the differences in service effectiveness caused by such organisational factors.

Finally, Soreff and Elkins (1977) describe a CMHC consultation service in a general hospital which leads to a 'more comprehensive service', for example to emergency patients, and also to more efficient use of staff time. This study would need to be repeated on a larger scale to examine the value of such programmes in encouraging coordination.

Targeting

Some programmes are 'targeting' their efforts to priority client groups, in order to facilitate the provision of a comprehensive service. The process of evaluating the impact of a service is more straightforward when the population and the needs to be served are clearly articulated. For further discussion of this subject the reader is referred to the section on 'target efficiency'.

There are no studies which systematically compare the range and continuity of services offered to clients served by a targeted service as opposed to one which aims to provide services to a wide range of individuals with mental health problems. Comprehensive coverage of a catchment area would require several complimentary targeted services which were highly coordinated. Bachrach (1980) amongst others has emphasised that since in general chronic clients are not being well served, the effective design of a programme will depend on the targeting of a specific population who have identified needs. She emphasises the point that each programme which targets a population should be seen as only part of the whole service system.

Allen (1986) studied responses to one of the key groups, the difficult to treat patient in long-term hospital care. If these patients are returned to the community then they can be expected to need services which are tailored to the kinds of problems identified by Allen. These problems include staff dissatisfaction in dealing with the withdrawal shown by psychotic patients, and the threat to teamwork posed by the violent or aggressive patient. Targeting specific groups cannot necessarily be assumed to lead to greater coordination between services, nor to greater continuity of care.

Catchments and sectorization

It has been suggested that providing services to a specific catchment area will better facilitate provision of the necessary range of services needed by the population and the coordination of the efforts of different agencies in the achievement of this goal.

Gittelman (1972) proposes that sectorization is one solution to the delivery of comprehensive and non-fragmented quality care. He defines a sector as a given area with a defined population for which a particular mental health team or teams has responsibility for providing all mental health services. The term 'catchment area' usually means the same thing i.e. the area from which a facility or targeted service draws it's clients.

Babigian (1977) examines the impact of catchmented CMHCs on utilisation of services. He uses areas both before and after the advent of CMHCS as their own controls and also makes between service comparisons, and comparisons with areas remaining centreless. The study shows increased utilisation by the poor and the young, but less impact on those with drug or alcohol problems, or the elderly.

Tischler et al (1972a; 1972b) find that catchmenting is associated with a higher volume of care, greater accessibility, improved service delivery to disadvantaged groups and more favourable clinical practices. They compared one group with access to a catchmented CMHC and one with access to a non-catchmented centre. The findings seem to indicate that catchmented services improve the level of provision to some clients with previously hidden problems.

Ozarin (1971) reports on the experience of visiting CMHCs in the U.S. and is of the opinion that staff assignment by geographical region rather than to a particular service leads to more flexible and economical services. She feel that divided responsibility for care increases the possibility of breakdown in the continuity of care. Lindholm (1983) also examine sectorization of psychiatric services, and find that services become more accessible, with more emphasis on day and out patient care after introduction of sectorised care. Continuity of care and patient satisfaction were high with no increase in costs.

There is a debate about the effects of catchmenting on mental health provision. There has been some suggestion that continuity may be encouraged, and that more people may be served (as we have outlined above) by catchmented services, but others have found that care remains 'patchy' (Abrams 1977) and far from comprehensive. Some people point to the inadequacy of the catchment concept in planning and delivering services because of the lack of congruity between the catchment area and the location of 'communities'. A major drawback of catchmented services is that they can rarely be comprehensive because they cannot provide, cost-effectively, for disorders of low incidence and prevalence. Catchmented services usually have to be backed up by specialist services serving a larger geographical area e.g forensic psychiatric services. This is what Bachrach (1982) had in mind when she argued for less emphasis upon the importance of 'locality', and suggested that an adequate range of care depends upon the co-operative working of various smaller targeted programmes within a service. We feel it is important to note that, in the studies reviewed here, sectorization and catchmenting are not synonymous with the provision of decentralised services (which often retain elements of central control over some aspects of service. For, instance budgetary control is not always decentralised.)

Needs assessment

The provision of services based on an assessment of the needs of an area or client group is closely allied to the concept of targeting services to serve particular needs, as discussed above. Needs assessment can lead to a clarity in planning and evaluation which facilitates service improvement and cross-service comparison (Kamis, 1979). Royse and Drude (1982) have defined needs assessment as akin to 'defining the problem', and is therefore essential to service planning and evaluation. (See evaluation chapter). In the UK, recent legislation recognises the importance of a comprehensive initial assessment for service users, and there is some possibility that services may be able to use this information to plan to meet needs in a more flexible and responsive way.

DeWitt Kay (1978) advocates social area analysis as a needs assessment method to aid programme planning and evaluation. MacDevitt & MacDevitt (1987) report on a needs assessment survey conducted in a rural area, by students using the telephone. Hagedorn (1976) and Schwab (1975) also describe several needs assessment techniques for the CMHC, (including the 'key informant' technique, the 'community forum', and the 'nominal group' approach). They claim these methods will enable centres to monitor the match of the existing services to community needs. (For a further consideration of needs assessment techniques, see the evaluation chapter).

There are no studies relating specifically to the increased coordination or comprehensiveness of services in programmes adopting a needs assessment technique in their planning processes.

The use of volunteers

Gaps in the provision of psychiatric services are often filled by volunteer provision. The inclusion of volunteers in the comprehensive range of services provided to clients depends on adequate coordination and liaison efforts.

Blows (1967) describes the Westminster Pastoral Foundation, which sees over 500 clients a week who, it is said do not differ significantly from those attending the local department of psychiatry. It appears to be serving a real need for counselling services for those who cannot find this in the Health Service, or afford private practice. Beitman (1982) also claims that pastoral centres and other voluntary provision reach a population untouched by psychiatry, and they should become an integral part of the service system. Morris (1980) describes a centre used by several groups of volunteers and finds that many people who could have benefited from the centre were not made aware of it's services.

The coordination of volunteers with other services has not been the subject of rigorous evaluation. In the care of the elderly the use of paid informal carers has been studied by Challis & Davies (1986), who confirm the necessity for a case manager to co-ordinate care across the voluntary, statutory and private sectors.

The use of volunteers and untrained staff has been widely encouraged, and even deemed as an essential component of a comprehensive service. A study of CMHC staffing patterns showed that in 80 centres 42% of full time staff positions were filled by non-professional mental health workers (Levenson 1970). Bennet (1976) advocates the use of low-paid and unpaid staff to take on major roles with patients with long term problems to save money during the expensive deinstitutionalisation process.

O'Donnell and George (1977) used volunteer staff to provide supportive and emergency telephone counselling services on a 24 hour basis, and found that if they were carefully trained and selected they could function as effectively as professional staff in a simulated study which assessed various dimensions of counselling effectiveness.

Genther (1974) is far less enthusiastic about the manning of community based 'hotlines' by volunteers. The study involved a role playing client calling ten hotlines. He concludes that all the lines function at a 'level that was less than helpful (based on a validated scale, rated by two trained listeners). He suggests that in the 'zeal toward innovative programs the quality of the service is overlooked'. Genther, and O'Donnell and George (1977) recommend that volunteers should be carefully selected and trained for the specific task.

Sobey (1970) has suggested that 90% of projects in the U.S. could not function without nonprofessionals, who plug the gaps in the services and also perform tertiary preventive work which was previously exclusively the territory of professional. Tarail (1980) has proposed that indigenous paraprofessionals are necessary in order to provide a comprehensive 'bio-psycho-social' model of care.

Even the advocates of the use of paraprofessional staff draw attention to its drawbacks. Sobey (1970) indicates some role, communication and status strains with the professional staff. Bartles et al (1975) conducted a questionnaire study aimed at the directors of CMHCs which also highlighted problems of inter-staff relations and role confusions which needed clarification Training obviously plays an important part in enhancing the effectiveness of nonprofessionals.

Case management (see also concluding chapter)

An important development in the provision of a coordinated service, and one which makes use of thorough assessment procedures combined with the amalgamation of resources from several agents, is the concept of 'case management'. There have been a number of papers reporting the use of this system in relation to elderly and mentally ill people (Caro,1981; Challis & Davies, 1986; Intagliata, 1982; Lamb, 1980; 1982; Ruchlin & Morris, 1983; Sherwood & Morris, 1983). Its proponents regard it as particularly suited to providing care in the community for people with long-term problems.

Care is provided through the individually planned combination of different sources of support, and the whole care package is overseen by a single 'case manager'. It is possible to combine private, voluntary and statutory sectors of care. In some examples of the approach the budget is also administered by the case manager. Individual assessment is emphasised and an attempt is made to meet the needs revealed , and to avoid simply fitting the client into the existing service system.

Johnson & Rubin (1983) consider that the approach is particularly suited to meeting the needs of mentally ill people, especially those with long term needs which require regular monitoring. An attempt to introduce case management has recently been attempted in Salford (Whitehead, 1987).

A skilled case manager would be able to see the early signs of deterioration in the client's circumstances and provide the stable relationship which is so often lacking. Case management relies on more than one mode of helping, combines practical and therapeutic forms of help, makes use of resources outside the statutory sector, and extends the responsibility for the costs of the service. This produces a quite different set of incentives for professional workers, particularly social workers. Of all the professionals at work in the community, social workers probably exhibit more of the skills necessary to undertake this role. The coordinating role which they often play is crucial to effective case management (Challis & Davies, 1986), they have access to local authority resources, and are sometimes adept at practical activity. The areas in which they would require to develop the quality of their skills is in assessment, formulation and review.

The problems which case management has to overcome to work effectively, are the need to be accountable for workers in more than one agency, the need to obtain budgetary control, and the need to have the active support of carers, volunteers, and other professionals.

Self help groups

Although there has been an increase in the range of services provided by self help groups, there is no consensus about how mental health professionals and self help groups should optimally interact.

We did not find any systematic evidence that self-help groups can be successfully integrated into a range of service provisions, although it is self-evident that they are meeting a need, often born out of dissatisfaction with existing services. Their existence may add to the comprehensive nature of service provision, but it might contribute to some duplication of services. In a recent visit to the USA we observed that when the attention of the Alliance for the Mentally Ill (AMI) was directed at the politicians responsible for services, rather than at the professional providers, they had greater impact.

Service guides

Feldman (1971) describe the use of an 'expediter' in CMHCs whose role was to ensure the coordination of organisational aspects of an individual's care, such as the ease of transfer of files and the monitoring of follow up appointments. The 'service guide' function of nonprofessionals was described by Raft et al (1976). In this case the worker was specifically concerned with the continuity of care provided to clients living in a rural community. The 'service guide' consulted with psychiatrist but handled 90% of crisis cases alone, monitored reactions to medication, provided transport and arranged help from other services if necessary. He was also involved in case finding. Because the service guide was withdrawn from the team, Raft et al were able to compare the period before removal with the period afterwards. The number of blacks who used the clinic decreased by 20%, referrals from nursing homes declined by 85%, and there were no referrals from the black nursing home. There was a 50% decrease in the number of elderly people and hospitalisation rates for schizophrenics rose by 30%. Ten of these patients said that inadequate drug intake was a factor in their hospitalisation and half of the families felt that hospitalisation could have been avoided if the service guide had still been visiting their homes. Return visits to services fell by 25%.

Under these particular circumstances the use of a paid non-professional appears to have had an effective and economical impact in providing service continuity and preventing some hospitalisations. This form of non-professional independent advocate /keyworker should be further investigated, particularly in the light of the increasing complexity of service provision in the community. It is worth noting, in passing, that what appeared to be the effective element of the work of the service guide, is regarded as part of the role of community psychiatric nurses in the UK. It might be possible for these tasks to be successfully undertaken by a non professional with some training. They are crucially important (particularly for patients with long-term problems) but tend to be regarded as 'unworthy' of professional time.

Community involvement in planning

A method of planning comprehensive services in the US was to involve local participants in the planning process (Greer and Greer 1984). A study by Flynn (1973) points to the problems of the use of community members in planning services, the main one being the question of representative participation. Participants in the planning process of comprehensive centres in Colorado between 1963 and 1969 tended to be of high income and educational levels. There was little evidence of the presence of the young, the old, minority or carer groups in the process. They did find that the community representatives had a useful knowledge of the needs of their own areas. How many representatives are necessary to acquire this knowledge of all 'areas' is not known.

Private care

Tonkin Boyd (1987) proposes that private care is creating a comprehensive service by occupying the holes in 'the market', and has arisen, like self help, because of the failure of local policies in caring for some clients.

There are few studies of comprehensiveness and coordination involving private provisions. Seigel et al (1983) suggested a greater degree of direct client contact occurred in private in patient facilities in the USA. There is also some evidence to suggest that private care is more acceptable to some clients (see relevant section, this volume). Although private care in the UK is growing there has been no systematic study of its effects on service coverage and continuity. Elderly people as a client group will be the first to be studied in this respect since both the absolute level of, and the growth in, provision of private care for elderly people far outstrips that for mentally ill people, and forms a substantial part of the care available. The number of elderly people in private old people's homes rose by half between 1978 and 1982. During the same period the growth in private care was roughly four times that in all other services.

Organisational issues

Mental hospitals

Retaining the large mental hospitals as the focus for the coordination of comprehensive care has been suggested as one organisational pattern. Most writers on the subject acknowledge the need for community services to complete the processes begun by hospital care. Amesbury (1983) summarises this view: "the most desirable mental health system is a comprehensive mental health system which encompasses and integrates the tenets of the community psychiatry program with those of the state in patient facilities". Amesbury suggests that community psychiatry could only be successful for 'some patients', and that the hospital has to form part of the comprehensive service to the catchment (see also Tantam, 1986). Tyrer (1985) has suggested a 'hive system' of care where workers leave the hospital to visit the local community. He is of the opinion that this system integrates the best features of both approaches, and that although 'small is beautiful' central coordination is essential.

Kidd (1967) advocated a 'modern role' for the mental hospital, which would provide the full range of treatments, encourage continuity of care between staff, have an 'open door' and liaise with G.Ps, employ team working and joint work with the local authority. This could just as easily be the list of aims for a community mental health centre service, illustrating the fact that similar aims may be achieved by different means.

At the same time Newton (1967) claimed that coordination in the community was a 'theoretically possible but bureaucratic illusion, to be much more readily attained in a specialist psychiatric hospital. The evidence for this is scant and later papers (Fiester et al 1975) have examined both the advantages and disadvantages of a hospital base. The advantages are heavily staff centred e.g ready access to other staff, easy recruitment and high staff morale because of easy access to the 'professional accoutrements' of workers, such as libraries, offices etc. The disadvantages are related to service quality and the difficulty of adequately serving all the needs of a catchment area from a hospital base.

Hoult (1986) suggests that care for schizophrenic clients cannot be comprehensive in terms of their various needs if it is hospital based and that one consequence is high recidivism rates (the latter point is discussed in the chapter on effectiveness). Okin (1983) has strongly argued that hospitals simply provide the wrong type of care, and that the need is for a fundamentally different system; he and others, particularly in the UK, are keen to avoid the 'warehousing' and the harmful effects associated with institutions. There is tendency to regard all institutions, but particularly large ones, as harmful, whereas in fact there is little or no evidence to suggest that size per se is the most important factor, and much evidence to support the view that the harmful effects of institutions derive mainly from the poor quality of care given to the residents (Huxley,1990).

Primary care teams

It is generally accepted that large numbers of people with psychiatric morbidity are supported by family doctors (Goldberg & Huxley, 1980), and that the general medical needs of psychiatric clients may be poorly served, as has already been discussed. There are problems relating to the appropriate referral of clients to the specialised services (Kessler 1977), and the continuity of care between the two systems; only 6% of people receiving care are getting services in both sectors (Regier et al 1978). The Presidents Commission on Mental Health (1978) also noted that co-operative working arrangements between the two sectors are rare, although there are a number of examples in the UK. These are described by Srathdee & Williams (1986) as the replacement model (in which the psychiatrist replaces the GP as the first point of contact), the increased throughput model (in which the GP refers a greater number of patients to the psychiatrist), and the liaison-attachment model. The last of these can be found in three patterns, the liaison-attachment 'team' pattern, in which the psychiatrist develops working relationships with other disciplines attached to the primary care team, the 'consultation' pattern, in which the psychiatrist saw the patient and advised the GP on management, and the 'shifted out-patient' pattern, which, although an alternative to an out-patient clinic appointment differed from it by the increased availability of background information about the patient and the participation of the GP in the assessment process.

This specific problem of service coordination leads calls for the integration of the primary care team and mental health care systems. Broskowski (1974) suggests that the integration of mental and physical health care delivery systems would be the best way to improve services. The training of medical personnel to recognise and manage patients with mental health problems has also been investigated (Goldberg & Huxley 1980). It may lead to the better serving of clients' needs, but it may not lead to the meeting of the needs of all clients, for example those who often underuse primary health care services, especially clients with long term problems.

Borus (1976) advocates neighbourhood health centres as the providers of mental health care to increase accessibility and acceptability, enhance case finding and aid successful coordination and referral. His suggestion includes coordination with the local CMHC to provide comprehensive care. In his view a specific person may have to adopt the role of integrating the efforts of health and mental health professionals.

Shepherd (1987) identifies some of the barriers which may have to be removed before this is possible. He sees the major barriers as the attitudes of clients to their health problems and the education and attitudes of G.Ps. A good deal of work has been done on improving G.P.s ability to detect minor psychiatric morbidity (Goldberg & Huxley,1980) and few people would now concur with Fink, who said 'I no longer believe that the GP can develop psychiatric skills'.

Primary care teams vary in their composition and there have been several attempts to study the nature of the service which results from the attachment of other professionals to the primary health care team. Corney (1980, 1984) studied the effects of attaching a social worker to a G.P practice. She found that clients referred to the scheme were more representative of the population of the area, and that cases were discussed with more agencies (60% discussed with the G.P and 20% with health visitors compared to 5% with the G.P for clients referred to social services area based workers). Huxley et al, in the results of a recent study, as yet unpublished, also found a high level of involvement between the GPs and attached social workers in the study. Area based social workers had almost no contact with GPs but had some contact with other team members, notably, the health visitor. In Corney's study attachment social workers tended to maintain contact when another agency was involved and area based social workers tended to relinquish it. It appears that such schemes may have an impact on the continuity of care for referred clients and may also lead to those with previously unserved mental health needs receiving care.

Corser and Ryce (1977) studied the attachment of a psychologist, a CPN and a sessional psychiatrist to a G.P. The referral rate to the psychiatrist doubled and communication between the professions increased. Common case notes were used. They suggest that the scheme enabled them 'to provide a full range of services' without recourse to hospital psychiatry, although in fact 16% of patients were admitted to the hospital.

Some papers relate specifically to the coordination between primary care teams and CMHC services (Goldman et al 1980). Florenzano (1977) suggest that G.Ps should be attached to CMHCs rather than the other way round. France (1978) found that only 10% of patients referred from primary care doctors to a CMHC actually completed referral indicating poor levels of coordination between the two. France suggested that G.Ps should personally seek to establish contact between the centre and the client rather than just advise it, in order to help the client to overcome any psychological barriers to access.

Perkins (1974) examines physicians attitudes towards CMHCs. Although 75% report a favourable attitude, only 20% use the centre and 50% have little or no knowledge about the centre or it's services. Some authors have argued that there is a need to examine the medical attitudes to psychiatric care and to attempt to remove any barriers to care which result from unhelpful attitudes.

Community Mental Health Centres

Much of the research relating to the coordination of a comprehensive service from a CMHC has already been described. Dowell and Ciarlo (1983) feel that better coordination is still needed between services, although the range and quantity of services had increased. Many centres were overwhelmed by the extent of the services which they were required to provide. Some authors show that the CMHC services, although aimed at underserved client groups, often failed to reach them, in a comprehensive way. A comprehensive service was not provided in relation to the needs of black clients (Armstrong, 1984) and lower socio-economic groups. Levin et al (1978) examined the relationship between services judged necessary by therapists and those actually received by clients in six CMHCs. Clients were deemed to be in need of an average of three services, but were offered only 1.6 . 21% were not rendered any service and 11% were not offered any service. Collaboration with other agencies on the clients' behalf occurred in 47% of the cases in which it had been recorded as necessary.

Dowell and Ciarlo (1983) estimate that 25 to 40% of clients drop out of treatment at CMHCs. Unfortunately they did not find any studies relating to interorganisational interactions but concentrated on within service features. Rothman and Kay (1982) specifically studied the relationship between CMHCs and family service agencies, which have many complimentary functions. They found that interrelations were far from optimal, and suggested that they need to be improved, although this need not involve a merging of services, merely closer cooperation.

Nuehring (1979) surveyed 30 CMHCs and found that interorganisational factors accounted for much of the variation in the type of consultation activities in which they were involved. For example, centres which encouraged organisational autonomy emphasised public education, whilst insular CMHCs concentrated on consultation by request. Urban centres focused on the training of other service providers. If interagency ties were extensive then more community planning and development emerged.

Jones (1979) clearly advocates the CMHC system as a means of integrating mental health services in the U.K. She stresses that the conceptual models underlying service delivery 'may make the difference between the encouragement or destruction of good psychiatric practice', and complains of the 'muddled policy thinking' which has lead to the current plethora of models in service provision. These models are plagued by unrealistic goals, and the split between several different bureaucratic authorities, leading to fragmented and unbalanced services.

Jones suggests that any successes in coordinating services in the past reflected a triumph over administrative adversities and was nearly thwarted by the insistence on 'medical confidentiality' of records. She also argues strongly that the family doctor does not have the resources to control the allocation of the new scattered services, since he/she does not have administrative responsibility for them or the training adequate to the task. This seems to be substantiated by the limited amount of research which we have found on the subject.

Mollica (1980) replied to Jones (1979), siting evidence that the elderly are not well served by CMHCs, and that the state hospitals remained important as a source of in patient care (because resources remained tied up in them?). He claims this indicates a failure to provide a comprehensive service which could meet all needs, although he agrees that catchmenting and out reach work may have improved services to minority groups. He also notes the reduced psychiatric presence in centres, the retreat to traditional treatment approaches, and the treatment of minority and lower class clients by low paid and often un-qualified staff.

Even if CMHCs can provide internally coordinated services for their clients, they still have to co-ordinate their efforts with district general hospitals, primary care teams, voluntary agencies and local authority services to provide a comprehensive, non duplicative service to all clients in their area. They will thus face the same problems of integration, which are caused by funding and planning problems as all the other service systems which have been proposed as the most appropriate 'focus' of mental health care in this country.

CMHCs cannot simply be assumed to remove the barriers to interagency communication which we have pointed out; i.e the problems of interprofessional interaction, interagency expectations, and services which are inappropriate or unacceptable to clients. It may be continual avoidance of these issues which leads to the circle of over-promise, under-production which Feldman (1979) describes as being characteristic of mental health provision and revolutions, and which are the consequences of 'faith' planning.

Introducing services systems which purport to remove all deficiencies of past service systems is blatantly misleading and harmful. Planning new services should be based on the evidence of the success or failure of specific aspects of service provision or on their strengths and weaknesses. This is probably the most important issue which must be addressed in the U.K. The ultimate attainment of the provision of coordinated and comprehensive mental health care to all those who are in need of it will have to start from this evidence, not from the incredible combination of an unquestioning acceptance of fashionable ideas and the total rejection of all past forms of care.

Summary and conclusions

1
Comprehensiveness and coordination are very widely accepted
service objectives (WHO 1977; R.C. Psychiat.1987; DHSS 1979)
and were an integral part of the CMHC mandate (Feldman,1979;
Dowell & Ciarlo, 1983; GAO, 1974). They are regarded as essential to the efficiency and effectiveness of services.
2
Conceptual confusion exists, in that 'comprehensive' often includes 'coordination' and vice versa.
3
Comprehensive can refer to a service for all the mental health
needs of a population, or all the needs of individual clients (i.e.
medical, psychosocial etc).
4
The term comprehensive, when used in relation to CMHCs
usually means the provision of the five essential services. These
are inpatient care, out-patient services, emergency services,
partial hospitalisation, and consultation & education.
5
Coordination usually refers to continuity of individual care.
The most common problem in the achievement of coordinated
services is client 'drop-out'. The reasons for client drop out could
include successful treatment, inappropriate services or their own
dissatisfaction. It is not clear which of these is of most importance in CMHC clients.
6
Among the CMHC service features which have been introduced
deliberately to improve coordination and/or extend service
coverage are: multidisciplinary teams; key workers; joint planning; consultation and education; targeting; catchments and
sectorization; needs assessment; the use of volunteers; self help
groups; service guides; community involvement in planning; and
private care. There is little evidence that any of these have actually resulted in more comprehensive or better coordinated care,
nor that they have improved outcome for clients.
7
Only sectorization and catchments appear to improve the coordination of care (Babigian, 1977; Lindholm, 1983 (Scandinavia);
Tischler, 1972).
8
There are a number of organisational issues which emerge as
important. Firstly the type of care provided by the mental hospital, especially for very disabled people with long-term needs, has
a place in the total service. Secondly, there are major coordination problems in primary health care. Thirdly, it is easier to
introduce services like CMHCs when there are no, or few, exist-

ing services. It is much more problematic to attempt to introduce new services where a lot of competing services already exist. In these circumstances new developments should have very clear target groups and clear service objectives.

9

There is considerable agreement that successful community services for people with long-term needs must have a range of available settings, including alternatives to institutional care, a person with clear responsibility for each client, and a degree of budgetary control (Aiken, 1988).

10

There have not been enough studies of the effect of different combinations of types of service, i.e. different professional groups, or mixtures of statutory and non-statutory services. Research into the differential effects of different 'input-mixes' is urgently needed. No such studies emerged from the CMHC literature.

References

Abrams, P. (1977) Community Care: Some Research Problems and Priorities. *Policy and Politics* 6:125-151.

Adler, P.T. (1977) The CMHC in the Community: Another Look. *Journal of Community Psychology* 5(2) p 166-123.

Aiken, L. (1988) Robert Wood Johnson program to evaluate care of serious mental illness. In Marks, I. Connolly, J. & Muijen, M. *New Directions in Mental Health Care Evaluation.* Institute of Psychiatry, London.

Albini, J.L. (1963) The Role of the Social Worker in an Experimental C.M.H. Clinic. *Community Mental Health Journal* 4(2):110-119.

Allen, J.G. (1986) Problems to anticipate in treating difficult patients in long term psychiatric hospital. *Psychiatry*, 49:350.

Amesbury, W.H. (1983) The comprehensive mental health system. *Perspectives in Psychiatric Care* 21(1):31-33.

Antinnen, E.E., Jokinen, R. & Ojanen, M. (1985) Progressive integrated system for rehabilitation of long term schizophren ic patients. *Acta Psych. Scand. Suppl.*319: (71):51-59.

Armstrong, H.E. et al (1984) Service utilization by black & white clients in urban C.M.H. *C.M.H. Journal* 20(4):269-81.

Babigian, H.M. (1977) The impact of CMHCs on the utilization of services. *Arch. Gen.Psychiat.* 34(4): 385-94.

Bachrach, L.L. (1980) Overview: Model Programmes for Chronic Mental Patients. *Am. Journal of Psychiatry* 137:9:1023-1031.

Bachrach, L.L. (1982) Assessment of Outcomes in Community Support Systems: Results, Problems and Limitations. *Schizo phrenia Bulletin* 8(1):39-57.

Bartles, B.D. et al (1975) Paraprofessionals in CMHCs. *Professional Psychology*, 6(4):442-52.

Bass, R. & Windle, C. (1972) Continuity of care: An Approach to measurement. *Am.J.Psych.* 129(2):196-201.

Beitman, B.D. (1982) Pastoral Counselling centers:A challenge to CMHCs. *Hosp. & Comm. Psych.* 33(6):486-7.

Belleck, A.S. & Meuser, K.T. (1986) A comprehensive treatment program for schizophrenia & chronic mental illness. *Comm. M.H. Journal* 22(3):175-190.

Bennett, D. (1976) Alternatives to Mental Hospital Treatment. *Hospital and Community Psychiatry* 27(3):186-92.

Bennett, D.(1978) Community Psychiatry. *Brit.J.Psych.* 132:209-20.

Birch, L. (1983) *What Chance Have We Got?* MIND, London.

Blaney, D. and West, A. (1987) Out of hours referrals to a general psychiatric hospital. *Health Bulletin* 45:67-70.

Bloom, B.L. (1976) Interdisciplinary Training: Attitudes and Practices in Community Mental Health. *Am.J.Orthopsychiat.* 46(4).

Blows, D. (1967) Westminster Pastoral Foundation. *Counselling*, 59:20-25.

Borus, J.F. (1976) Neighbourhood health centers as providers of primary health care. *New England J.Med.* 295:140-145.

Broskowski, A. & Baker,F. (1974) Professional, Organisational & social barriers to primary prevention. *Am.J. Orthpsych.* 44(5):707-719.

Burgoyne, R.W. et al (1979) Patients Requests of an Outpatient Clinic. *Arch. Gen. Psychiat.* 36:400-403.

Caro, F.G. (1981) Demonstrating community based long term care in the US: An Evaluation Perspective. In Goldberg & Connolly, *Evaluating Research in Social Care*. Heinemann, London.

Challis, D. & Davies, B. (1986) *Case Management in Community Care*. Gower, Aldershot.

Cline, H.F. & Sinnott, L. T. (1981) What can we learn about change in organisations? In Ball, *New Directions for Program Evaluation*.

Corney, R.H. (1980) Comparative Study of Referrals to a L.A.Intake Team. *Soc. Sci. and Med.* 14A:675-682.

Corney, R.H. (1984) Effectiveness of attached social workers in the management of depressed female patients. *Psych. Med.Suppl* 6:1-46.

Corser, C.M. & Ryce, L. (1977) Community mental health care - a model based on the primary care team. *B.M.J.* 2(i):936-938.

Cowen, E. (1978) Some Problems in Community Program Evaluation Research. *J.Consult.Clin.Psych.* 46:792-805.

Creer, C. & Wing, J.K. (1974). *Schizophrenia at home*. National Schizophrenia Fellowship, Surbiton.

DeWitt Kay, F. (1978) Applications of Social Area Analysis to Program Planning & Evaluation. *Eval.& Prog. Planning* 1:65-78.

Donovan, C.M. (1982) Problems of Psychiatric Practice in CMHCs. *Am.J.Psych.* 139(4):458-460.

Dowell, D.A. & Ciarlo, J.A. (1983) Overview of the C.M.H.C. Program from an Evaluation Perspective. *Comm.M.H.Journal* 19:95-125.

Erbinger, R. & Christy Brown (1980). Social deprivation amongst short stay hospital patients. *Brit. J.Psychiat.* 136:46-52.

Eysenck, S. (1987) Mentally Disordered Individuals in the Prison System. *Just. Peace.* April, 25:265.

Feldman, S. (1971) Ideas and issues in community mental health. *Hosp. & Comm. Psych.* 22(11):17-21.

Feldman, S. (1978) Promises, promises or Community Mental Health Services and Training: Ships that pass in the night. *Comm.M.H.Journal* 14(2).

Feldman, S. (1979) CMHCs in the US. *J.R. Soc.Med.* 72:633-634.

Fiester, A.R., Silverman, W.H. & Beech, R.P. (1975) Problems involved in delivering emergency services in hospital based CMHCs. *J.Comm.Psychol.* 3(2):188-192.

Fink, E.B. et al (1979) Examination of clinician bias in patient referrals in partial hospitalization settings. *Hosp.Comm. Psych.* 30(9):631-32.

Florenzano, R. & Raft, D. (1977) How best to utilise your CMHC. *N.Carolina Med. J.* 38(4):206-8.

Flynn, J.P. (1973) Local Participants in Planning for Comprehensive CMHCs. *Comm.M.H. Journal* 9(1):3-10.

Foley, H.A. & Sharfstein, S.S. (1983) *Madness and Government: WhoCares for the Mentally Ill?*. American Psychiatric Press, Washington D.C.

France, R.D. et al (1978) Referral of patients from primary care physicians. *J.Nerv.Ment. Dis.* 166:594-598.

Freeman, H. (1976) Continuity of care in a mental health service *Int.J.Ment.Health* 5:3-13.

Genther, R. (1974) Evaluation of the functioning of community based hotlines. *Prof.Psych.* 5:409-414.

Gilleard, C.J. (1987) Influence of emotional distress among supporters on the outcome of psychogeriatric day care. *B.J. Psych.* 150:219-223.

Gittleman, M. (1972) Sectorization:The Quiet Revloution in European Mental Health Care. *Am.J.Orthopsych.* 42(1):159-167.

Glasscote, R.M. (1969) *The CMHC - An Interim Appraisal.* Washington Joint Information Service of the APA and NAMH.

Goldberg, D. & Huxley, P. (1980) *Mental illness in the Community* Tavistock, London.

Goldberg, D., Kay, C. & Thompson, L. (1976) Psychiatric morbidity in general practice and the community. *Psych. Med.* 6:565-69.

Goldman, H.H. et al (1980) Integrating primary health care and mental health services. *Pub. Health Report* 95(6):535-539.

Grad, J.C. (1968) A Two Year Follow-Up. In Williams, R.H. & Ozarin, L.D. *Community Mental Health.* Jossey Bass, San Francisco.

Greer, S. & Greer, A.L. (1984) The Continuity of Moral Reform *Soc. Sci. & Med.* 19(4):397-404.

Griffith, J.H. & Mangen, S.P. (1980) Community Psychiatric Nursing - a literature review. *Int. J.Nurs. Stud.* 17:197-210.

Gruber, L.N., Brown, A. & Mazorol, C. (1978) Ex-patient Visitors to the Hospital Psychiatric Unit. *Hosp.Comm.Psychiat.* 29(1):731-734.

Hagedorn, H. J. et al (1076) *A working Manual of Simple Program Evaluation Techniques for CMHCs.* NIMH DHEW Publication No (ADM) 76-404.

Harakal, C. (1975) An Instrument to assess Staff Time Utilization in CMHCs. *Comm.M.H.Journal* 11(4):371-380.

Haw, C. (1987) Patients at a psychiatric walk in clinic. *Bulletin of the R.C. Psych.*

Henderson, J.G. (1973) Role of the Psychiatric Nurse in a Domicilliary Treatment Service. *Nursing Times* 18:1377-8.

Hodges, A. & Mahoney, S.C. (1970) Expectations for the comprehensive CMHC. *C.M.H. Journal* 6(1).

Hoshall, D. & Freidman, J. (1975) Evaluation from a former patient's point of view. *Evaluation* 2(2):8-9.

Hunt, L.B. (1983) Community Services for Community Care.*Health Trends* 15:77-81.

Hunter, P. (1980) Social Work and Community Psychiatric Nursing *Int.J.Nurs.Studs.* 17:131-139.

Huntingdon,J. (1981) *Social Work & General Medical Practice: Collaboration or conflict?* George Allen & Unwin, London.

Huxley, P.J. (1990) The sociology of size in residential care. In M.Davies & D.Howe *The Sociology of Social Work*, Gower, Aldershot.

Intagliata, J. (1982) Improving the Quality of Community Care: the role of case management. *Schizophrenia Bulletin* 8(4):655-674.

Johnson, P.J. Rubin, A. (1983) Case management in mental health: a social work domain? *Social Work* 281:49-56.

Jones, K. (1979) Deinstitutionalisation in context. *Mill. Mem. Fund. Quarterly* 57(4):552-569.

Kamis, E. (1979) A Witness for the Defense of Needs Assessment.*Evaluation & Program Planning* 2(1):7-12.

Keith, S.J. (1978) Community Support Systems:Multifactorial Approaches to complex problems. *Schizophrenia Bulletin* 4(3):316-7.

Kessler, L.G. et al (1977) Psychiatric Diagnosis of Medical Services Users. *Am.J.Pub.Health* 18-24.

Kidd, H. (1967) Modern Role of the Psychiatric Hospital. In Freeman, H. & Farndale, J. (eds) *New Aspects of the Mental Health Services*. Permagon, Oxford.

Lamb, H.R. (1980a) Structure the Neglected Ingredient in Community Psychiatry. *Arch. Gen. Psych.* 37:1124-27.

Lamb, H.R. (1980b) Therapist case-managers: more than brokers of services. *Hosp. & Comm. Psych.* 31:14-18.

Lamb, H.R. (1982) *Treating the long-term mentally ill.* Jossey Bass, London.

Lancaster, J. (1980) *Community mental health nursing - an ecological Perspective.* C.V. Mosby, London.

Lang, C.L. (1982) Isolation of status and ideological conflicts in a CMH setting. *Psych.* 45:159-171

Langsley, D.G. (1975) Community Mental Health: A Review of the Literature. In Barton,W.E.& Sanborn, C.J. *An Assessment of the CMHC Movement.* Lexington , Mass.

Leaf, P.J. (1985) Contact with health professionals for treatment of psychiatric problems. *Med.Care* 23(12):1322-37.

Leong, G.B. (1982) Psychiatrists and CMHCs. *Hosp. & Comm Psych.* 33(4): 309-11.

Levenson, A.I. & Reff, S.R. (1970) CMHC Staffing Patterns.*Comm.M.H. Journal* 6(2):118-125.

Levin,G., Wilder, J.F. & Gilbert, J. (1978) Identifying and meeting client's needs in six CMHCs. *Hosp. & Comm. Psychiat.* 29(3).

Lindholm, H. (1983) Sectorized Psychiatry. *Acta Psychiat. Scand.* (Suppl. 304) 67:1-127.

Littlewood, R. (1986) *Psychiatric Services for Black and other Minority Groups in Birmingham.* Paper for the workshop 'Providing Acceptable Services for Black and Minority Ethnic groups'. July 7.

Maisey, M.A. (1975) Hospital Based Psychiatric Nurses in the community. *Nursing Times.* Feb 27:354

MacDevitt, M. & MacDevitt, J. (1987) Low cost Needs Assessment for a Rural Mental Health Center. *J. of Counselling & Development* 65(9):505-507.

Mollica, R.F. (1980) CMHC - American Response to Kathleen Jones *J.Roy.Soc.Med.* 73:6863-870.

Morris, P. (1980) Working for health in Sheffield. *Mind Out* 38:24.

Murray, J.E. (1975) Failure of the community mental health movement. *Am.J.Nursing* 75:11.

Nuehring, E.M. (1979) Preventive activity and interoganisational factors. *J.Soc.Service Research* 2(3):285-300.

O'Donnell, J.M. & George, K. (1977). Use of volunteer in a CMHC *Comm.M.H.Journal* 13 (1):3-9.

Okin, R.L. (1983) Future of state hospitals. *Am.J.Psych.* 145(5):577-81.

Ozarin, L. (1971) Experience with CMHCs. *Am. J. Psychiat.* 27(7):912.

Pepper, B. & Ryglewicz, H. (1982) Unified Services: Concept and Practice. *Hosp.Comm.Psychiat.* 33(9):762-765.

Perkins, D.V. (1974) An assessment of physicians' attitudes towards Community Mental Health. *Comm.M.H. Journal* 10(3):282-91.

Raft, D.D. et al (1976) Using a service guide to provide comprehensive care in a rural CMHC. *Hosp. & Comm. Psych.* 27(8):553-9.

Regier, D., Goldberg, I.D. & Taube, C. (1978) The De Facto US Mental Health Services System: A Public Health Perspective *Arch.Gen.Psychiat.* 35:685-693.

Reich, R., & Seigel, L. (1973) Chronically mentally ill shuffle to oblivion. In Freedman, et al. *Psychiatry under siege.*

Reich, R. (1973) Care of chronically mentally ill. *Am.J.Psychiat.* 130(8):911-12.

Reinstein, M.J. (1978) CMHCs & The dissatisfied psychiatrist: an informal survey. *Hosp. & Comm. Psychiat.* 29(40:261.

Rothman, J. & Kay, T. (1982). CMHCs and Family Service Agencies *Soc. Wk. Research & Abstracts* 10:16.

Royal College of Psychiatrists (1987). *A Carer's Perspective* R.C.P., London.

Royse, D. & Drude, K. (1982). Mental health needs assessment: beware of false promises. *Comm.M.H.Journal* 18(2):97-106.

Ruchlin, H.S. & Morris, J.H. (1983). Pennsylvania's Domiciliary Care Experiment II:Cost benefit implications. *Am.J.Pub. Health.* 736:645-660.

Sayce, L. (1987). *CMHCs Conference Report.* National Unit for Psychiatric Research & Development, London.

Schrameijer, F. (1987). New Comprehensive Mental Health Authorities in the Netherlands. *Int.J.Soc.Psychiat.* 33(2):132-136.

Schulberg, H.C. & Bromet, E. (1981). Strategies for evaluation of community services for chronically mentally ill *Am.J.Psych.* 138(7):930-935.

Schwab, et al (1975). An epidemiological assessment of needs and utilisation of services. *Evaluation* 2(2):65-67.

Sharfstein, S. (1978) Will Community Mental Health Survive in the 1980's? *Am.J.Psychiat.* 135(11):1363-1365.

Shepherd, M (1987). Mental illness and primary care. *Am.J.Pub.Health* 12-13.

Sherwood, S. & Morris, J.N. (1983). The Pennsylvania Domiciliary Care Experiment I:Impact on Quality of Life *Am.J.Pub. Health* 736:646-653.

Siegel, C. et al (1983). Comparison of work activities of mental health professionals. *Hosp.Comm.Psych* 34(2):154-157.

Skuse, D. Williams, P. (1984). Screening for psychiatric disorders in geneal practice. *Psych. Med.* 14:365-77.

Sobey, F. (1970). *The non-professional revolution in mental health.* Colombia University Press.

Social Services Select Committee (1985). 2nd Report, *Community Care with special reference to adult mental illness.* HMSO, London.

Soreff, S.M. & Elkins, A.M. (1977). A CMHC Consultation service in a general hospital. *Hosp. & Comm Psychiat.* 28 (10):749-753.

Specht, D.I. (1983). Study of employees in transition from hospital to community programs. *Hosp. & Comm. Psychiat.* 28 (10):749-753.

Stelovich, S. (1979). From hospital to prison. *Hosp. & Comm.Psychiat.* 30(9):618-20.

Strathdee, G. & Williams, P. (1984). Patterns of collaboration In Shepherd, M. *Mental Illness in Primary Care Settings.*

Tantam, D. (1986). Alternatives to psychiatric hospitalisation *Brit.J.Psychiat.*146: 1-4.

Tarail, M. (1980). Current and future issues in community mental health. *Psychiat. Quart.* 52 (1):27.

Test, M.A. & Stein, L.I. (1980). Alternative to mental hospital treatment. *Arch.Gen.Psychiat.* 37:409-412.

Test, M.A. & Stein, L.I. (1978) Training in Community Living: Research design and results. In Stein, L.I. & Test, M.A. (Eds) *Alternatives to Mental Hospital Treatment.* Plenum Press, New York.

Test, M.A. (1981). Effective community treatment of the chronically mentally ill. *J.Soc. Issues* 37(3).

Tischler, G.L., Henisz, J., Myers, J.K. & Garrison, V. (1972a) Catchmenting and the use of mental health services.*Arch.Gen. Psychiat.* 27:389-392.

Tischler, G.L., Henisz, J., Myers, J.K. & Garrison, V. (1972b) The impact of catchmenting. *Admin. in Mental Health*, Winter:22-29.

Tonkin, B. (1987). Is private care better care? *Community Care* April: 23-25.

Towell, D. & McAusland, T. (1984). Managing Psychiatric Services in Transition. *Health & Social Services Journal* Oct 25:1-8.

Tryer, P. (1985). The Hive System. *Brit. J. Psychiat.* 146:571-575.

Whitehead, C. (1987). *Care of long term psychiatric patients.* Salford District Health Authority.

Wooff, K. (1986) A Comparison of roles of CPN's and PSW's.*Ph.D. Thesis* University of Manchester, Department of Community Medicine.

Williams, R.H. (1968). Major Issues. In Williams & Ozarin *Community Mental Health*, New York, Jossey Bass.

Wistow, G. (1987). Joint finance:promoting a new balance of care in England? *Int. J.Soc.Psychiat.* 33(2):83-91.

Yamanoto, J. (1984). Orienting therapists' and patients' needs to increase patient satisfaction. *Am.J.Psychiat.in.Med* 9:339-350.

Zusman, J. & Slawson, M. (1972). Service quality profile. *Arch. Gen. Psychiat.* 27:692-98.

Zusman, J. (1975). Philosophic basis for a community and social psychiatry. In Barton & Sanborn. *op. cit.*

3 Accessible and acceptable services

Introduction

There is considerable evidence that health care resources are unevenly distributed, so that people who are thought to be most in need often receive a lower proportion of resources than they merit. Hart (1971) has termed this "inverse care law". In the absence of evidence to the contrary (Macintyre, 1986) many people simply assume that improved access will lead to improvement in the distribution of health care and an improvement in outcome.

As one of the main goals of the CMHC movement in the USA, accessibility has received a good deal of attention. It is a multi-faceted concept which requires clarification (Holland,1975). A major problem is the way in which several different concepts are nested within one global concept of accessibility. We located the following meanings of accessibility and acceptability in the literature. We have subdivided these into major categories, around which we structure the remainder of this section. An accessible service is one which is:

Geographically accessible
>   physically near to clients homes
>   entails little travel and inconvenience
>   available in all areas
>   dispersed from a central site
>   utilised by all groups in the locality

Bureaucratically accessible
>easy to gain entry to
>presents no unnecessary barriers to care
>maximally available for use around the clock
>not dependent on the vagaries of gate keepers
>offers minimal delay to clients
>which has straightforward referral procedures
>caters for those inadequately served elsewhere
>allows entry to alternative forms of care groups
>does not exercise preferential selection

Cognitively accessible
>visible (known about) to those in need
>whose whereabouts is widely known
>whose role and functions are well understood

Psychologically accessible or acceptability
>initially appealing to those in need
>initially not threatening to clients self esteem
>attracts those who traditionally avoid services
>perceived as less/non stigmatising to clients
>perceived as welcoming, homely or friendly
>avoids the worst aspects of institutional appearance
>whose role and functions are well accepted
>appropriate to client' perceived need
>provides an equitable service to all
>not judgmental in respect of client's needs
>delivered by competent people

We will be referring to the several different aspects of accessibility in the remainder of this chapter. The aspect most frequently found in the literature is geographic accessibility, or proximity. There are several other equally important aspects, which are: cognitive (do people know where the service is, what it is for, who is eligible, and how to access it?); bureaucratic (is there a referral system, is there a waiting list etc.?) and psychological. The last of these is synonymous with acceptability (is it the sort of service which the person wants, likes and is satisfied with?). In order for a service to be accessible it has, by definition, to be available. For instance, an emergency service should be part of a total service coverage.

Availability does not exist if the service is not part of the total service coverage. If a service is part of the total service coverage but is denied to the individual in need of it, then it is available, but inaccessible. As already indicated, there can be several different reasons why an available service remains inaccessible.

From this introduction it is clear that accessibility of services is a complex matter. If one is unclear about the reasons for the non or under use of a service then one may make mistakes in attempting to improve access. For instance, if the main problem with access to services, is their absence in certain areas, the difficulty of travelling to remote sites, or lack of knowledge of the availability of a service, then a highly visible and locally promoted mental health service may be ideal. However, if underuse of mental health services is caused by potential clients' fears of stigma, then a highly visible and locally promoted mental health service may not be ideal.

A less obvious problem is the possibility that a strategy which may make a service attractive to one group of clients, may not make it attractive to another. The use of a service by one group may lead to underuse by other groups, especially if one group is regarded as socially unattractive by the other.

Service strategies aimed at improving access

The following service delivery strategies are all identified in the literature as ways in which the CMHC movement attempted to improve access to services.

localising services
providing smaller units/ more personal
around the clock cover
use of volunteers
use of ethnic minority staff
use of "poor" staff
siting services in "poor" areas
siting services in minority areas
siting services in all areas
advertising/publicising services
increasing availability of care/more staff/more units
outreach to underserved groups
open door
extending self referral
abandoning initial appointments
educating public about mental health
educating prominent community members about mental health
providing free care
providing sliding fees
specially designed services for special groups
provision of native language speakers
locating unmet need in locality
evaluating and disseminating the performance of centres
changing the image of services
provision of a wider range of services
use of ordinary housing as sites of care

There is evidence to indicate that some of these strategies were effective to some extent in increasing the accessibility of services to some groups. Firm evidence for the relative efficacy of each of them is hard to find; that which does exist is reviewed below.

Availability

Service coverage

CMHCs partially achieved one of their major objectives, in that services were brought to some areas where previously there had been none (Ozarin 1971). NIMH data show that the provision of CMHCs clearly had an effect on the availability of services. When appropriately matched catchment areas, with and without federally funded centres are compared, over time (1973 and 1980), more people were being reached in those areas served by Centres (Windle et al 1987). It is well known that the creation of additional services generates a disproportionate increase in demand, (Rumer 1978, reviews numerous studies which show that this occurs when there is an increased supply of services). There has been considerable debate about whether the increase in use was mostly by people with minor rather than major mental illnesses. This is discussed later, but for the moment we can say that while there was an increase in use by people with minor disorders, there was also an increase in use by people with major disorders.

Service coverage in priority areas

In the USA, priority was initially given to the funding of CMHC's in poverty areas, and in summarising the evidence, Dowell & Ciarlo (1983) note that by 1975, 60% of all funded centres were in the poorer areas, even though finance to match federal funding was more difficult to acquire in these areas.

The 1977 NIMH report showed that this preference was not maintained however, so that although nearly all centres which received distress funds to keep them going were in poverty areas, by 1977 only half of all the funded centres were in poverty areas.

There is some indication that the funded centres were also situated preferentially in those areas where there were higher concentrations of ethnic minorities, but this was not a consistent pattern. There were also inadequacies in the siting of services in rural areas. Contrary to intentions, rural areas were less well served in terms of the number of funded centres and also manpower.

Availability of community services

However, in terms of service coverage the aim of CMHC legislation, (and of UK and Italian legislation among others) has been to provide community services rather than mental hospital services. The extent to which primary health care physicians dealt with major and minor psychiatric morbidity was not appreciated (by policy makers) at the time of the enactment of the CMHC legislation.

The CMHC mandate improved coverage but it was not until later that the de facto mental health service (the extent to which family physicians dealt with mental health problems) was revealed (Regier et al, 1978). In this important respect the USA and the UK are remarkably similar (Shepherd 1987). In respect of specialist service coverage there are similarities too, in that mental hospitals still provide care, DGH units in general hospitals provide care, and there is private care. While the UK has reasonable overall service coverage, there are substantial differences between regions, for instance in terms of manpower. Local authority services are immensely variable, and more importantly, are not mandatory. Even the specialist mental health manpower in local authorities (the approved social workers) are mandated without any guidance as to the appropriate numbers needed; this is left to the authority to decide.

The major difference between the USA and the UK, and indeed between the UK and most other western countries, was the way health care provision used to be funded. The pattern of service availability and use in the UK was, until recently, more or less entirely dependent upon the administration of NHS funds. The pattern is now changing, and the introduction of private care, private health insurance, health maintenance organisations (HMOs) and the like, will change patterns of availability and use, particularly in the specialist sector. Primary care may be less affected. The fear is that some areas will get many competing services and others will get none (du Sautoy 1987).

Regional and local inequalities in the availability of health services abound, even in the UK (Townsend & Davidson, 1982) and equal access to care is an ideal rather than a reality. The CMHCs were an attempt to increase availability to those groups who are traditionally underserved. In the next section we look at the extent to which they were able to take up the services on offer.

Availability to priority groups

If services are more accessible to priority groups then one would expect them to use the services more than less accessible services. This would produce higher utilisation rates per head of (priority group) population and a larger proportion of the total service users would be from the priority groups. In terms of efficiency, these coincide with horizontal and vertical target efficiency, respectively (see efficiency chapter).

There are several reasons why a simple judgment about the accessibility of CMHC services cannot be made. The main one is the great variability between centres. The proportion of the service used by known priority groups varies from none, in some cases, to all, in others. Rothman and Kay (1982), document this massive variability across centres. In terms of serving the poor the range across centres was from 10% to 96% of centre case loads; for schizophrenia the range was from 0% to 100%; for alcoholism from 0% to 47% ; for non-psychotic disorders, 0% to 67%; and for no mental disturbance from 0% to 98%.

Lower socio-economic groups

A comparison of inpatient characteristics across four services (private mental hospital, public mental hospital, CMHC and general hospital) showed that, in 1971, the state mental hospitals were still dealing with the highest percentage of the lower socio-economic groups, in comparison to CMHC's and private facilities (62%, 53% and 33%) (Ozarin 1974). More recent evidence reports as many as 90% of some state hospital patients come from low socioeconomic backgrounds (Derisi et al 1983).

A more extensive comparison period 1950-1975 (Mollica 1980) of utilisation rates across facilities, showed that low status patients were still to be found in excessive and unrepresentative numbers in state hospitals.

Ethnic minorities

Rosen et al (1980), in documenting the utilisation patterns in a centre located in a very poor area serving a culturally diverse population, (clients were predominantly from the lowest social status groupings, 92% lower social class, and 71% from ethnic minority groups) found that of the 87% admissions scheduled for follow up care, 12% of clients were consuming over 60% of the centres services. This was calculated in terms of total resources utilisation estimates (TRUE scores), and showed that diagnosis was the main factor responsible for most of the total variance, due to the high levels of usage by those with the most severe diagnoses.

Some authors have reported that the treatments offered varied by social group. Mollica (1980) argued that clients from lower status groups, when found in out patient care at Centres, tended to be on low status, low intervention programs, where the quality of care was regarded as inferior. Hart (1972) shows that there were systematic differences to be found in both the type of treatment and the amounts of staff time offered to clients of lower status ethnic minority clients. Armstrong (1984) finds similar conclusions in many studies, and in addition shows that even though black clients were significantly less impaired than white clients, they were given equivalent diagnostic labels but received fewer services. The more desirable and staff intensive types of care were disproportionately reserved for higher status clients.

Comparison of admissions to all sources of care by Ozarin (1974), showed that ethnic minority clients were not enjoying equal, access to all care options. Public mental hospitals and CMHC's were admitting the highest percentages (22% and 21% respectively), whilst both the general hospital and private care show markedly lower percentages, 16% and less than 5% respectively. In the UK concern has been expressed about the high rates of involuntary admission to mental hospitals of ethnic minority clients, the rate currently being three times that for white people (Littlewood 1986).

There is considerable evidence to indicate that both black and white lower socio-economic group clients are the least well served by provision in the US, and this applies to physical health care services as well as mental health care services. Goodman (1979), in a study which allowed for the investigation of the differential effects of social status and minority group membership on utilisation rates found that, although in the areas they studied, black clients sought services in greater numbers and at much higher rates than white clients, (9.5 and 2.3 per 1000 pop respectively),in terms of the average number of visits they made, lower social class black clients received treatment at significantly lower rates than lower class white clients. Black and white middle class clients received services at equal rates. Those least likely to seek care as a group (in this locality) were the lower status white clients, who nevertheless when in care tended to have very high rates of usage of long term care, mostly as inpatients.

Severe disorders

The severity of disorder treated in CMHCs seems to be intermediate in severity between public hospital and private practice patients. Their clientele appear to be most similar to that seen in public out patient clinics. In comparison to state hospitals, CMHC clientele appear to be less impaired, and they treat fewer people with alcohol problems, organic brain syndromes, and schizophrenia.

There have been many complaints about the CMHC's shifting away from the treatment of the most severely disabled towards the less severe "problems of living" (Dowell & Ciarlo, 1983; Borus 1978; Langsley, 1980; Bachrach, 1984; Phillips et al, 1981; Dorwart 1983; Phillips et al, 1976). Evidence was derived from such indicators as the falling proportions of those diagnosed with severe disorders in CMHC care, and the rising proportion of those without any specific mental disorder (see Target Efficiency for a more detailed discussion of these points). Pardes (1983) and

Dowell & Ciarlo (1983) point out that the trend was not uniform across all CMHC's, and that the older established CMHC's did not show the same tendency. Recent work suggests that psychiatrists in CMHCs tend to see more severely ill patients than do other professional groups (Windle et al, 1988a; 1988b).

Brown (1984) notes the great variability across centres in respect of the proportion of chronically ill clients seen. The proportion ranged between 10% and 70% of centre caseloads. Springer (1977) found that rates of acceptance for care varied considerably across centres and those without a specific diagnosis were the most likely to be rejected and considered to be "welfare problems". Level of education was significantly associated with the type of treatment offered in over half of the centres. Overall, the number of sessions on offer was low, 62% received up to three, 24% up to ten, and only 11% received more than ten.

Levin et al (1978) examined the extent to which a number of centres actually offered the services staff thought their clients required. On average clients were judged to need three services, of which only 1.6 were rendered. Fewer services were offered than planned, and not all of those offered were taken up. When one looks at the range of scores rather than the means, a great deal of variance is revealed. At one centre e.g. 51% of clients were rendered no service at all.

While there is little comparable evidence in the UK to date, changes in the level of private care for elderly people are already producing unequal access to residential services for lower income groups (Walker 1988). The CMHCs were unable to make any permanent, comprehensive improvement in access for lower income groups in the USA . The vast increases in professional and voluntary manpower which accompanied the development of CMHCs in the USA, are unlikely to be replicated in the UK. (Although 18000 psychiatric nurses might become available to work in the community if all the mental hospitals in the UK were to be closed, there are likely to be only 8,000 jobs available for them). Availability is unlikely to improve because of a manpower expansion, and access for priority groups is likely to diminish if the ability to pay (for services or insurance) becomes a more prominent feature of UK health care.

Geographic accessibility

Proximity

The geographic aspect of accessibility has received the most attention and seems to be the key meaning of the term in popular usage. Local services with small catchment areas are recommended as the best means "to get close to the people in need" (Gorman 1976; Bratcher 1977). The post-Barclay report service developments in the UK, including the concept of 'patch teams' and neighbourhood offices, is based on a good number of untested ideas and assumptions. Many of the resulting services are confused about the precise reasons for the creation of a 'local' service. Challis & Ferlie (1986) have usefully described the range of resulting organisational consequences in social services departments.

An important feature of geographic accessibility is the ease of travel to and from care. White (1987) looked at the effect of travel distance between clients' homes and the CMHC on the length of their use of services, and found them to be related. In another study the distance to be travelled was related to use (Hagedorn 1976). However Brandon in a more sophisticated study (1975) found that certain groups would make use of services whilst others would not, regardless of how close they were. Brandon found that social characteristics of clients were the main determinants of uptake, regardless of the siting of services. Some clients will travel to utilise services regardless of where they are provided, whilst others will ignore the services even if they are nearby. In a study in New Zealand, Hall (1988) found that distance did affect use of suburban centres, but did not affect the use of urban ones.

Orden & Sticking (1971) reported that staff in decentralised services thought that accessibility was improved by going local. No evidence that this was actually the case was provided. The results were obtained by asking staff at nine CMHCs for their opinions about the effects of the service on access, rather than by studying actual utilisation rates. Low income groups seemed to have improved access because local agencies were more likely to refer them.

The assumption that the mere siting of services locally will improve utilisation rates for all client groups is clearly an oversimplification. It overlooks the equally and in some respects more important aspects of accessibility which need to be considered. It would not be unreasonable to suppose that people prefer to use a service which is slightly further away, if it provides what they want more effectively, more efficiently, or, more simply, at times when they can use it.

Studies of the extent to which proximity is vital are lacking (Abrams 1977). No study has been conducted in an area which has similar and competing services to see whether geographical proximity is the key determinant of use, and what part the nature and cost of travel has on usage. In fact, the degree of conviction that providing services locally improves access would appear to be inversely related to the amount of evidence that it does so. Socio-economic factors are important determinants of use in the USA, where there are financial barriers to some forms of care, and socio-economic factors will be increasingly important in the UK if financial barriers to care become more common.

Bureaucratic accessibility

Filtering

The filtering of clients will be considered in some detail as both official and unofficial filtering of wanted and unwanted clients is an important determinant of accessibility (a bureaucratic means of selectively supplying services).

One study of the filtering process observed in one Centre will be reported in some detail here. Lang (1981) conducted a participant observation study over 18 months of the process of "warding off" unwanted clients in a centre which was part of a health service setting. The mental health centre staff (MHCS) had an educational role towards the health centre staff (HCS), and resisted the tendency of the latter to send difficult patients straight to them. Referrals to the MHCS came predominantly from the HCS and other units in the practice (20% were self referred, 25% from outside agencies, and 50% from HCS).The HCS had become very adept at case finding in their practice, and the MHCS had to hold back a flood of clients.

The MHCS also kept their links with the local welfare department to a minimum in order to 'ward off' difficult clients. Among the self referred clients, there were a number of chronic "perpetual cases", who were not assigned to a worker for treatment. Clearly, in this centre, some clients were systematically deflected from the service system. The author suggests the staff lacked specific training in dealing with the wide variability of clients requiring care, and they had not developed any new ways of working to cope with such demand.

In one review of the literature documenting the acceptance by staff of clients for therapy, Cobb (1972) notes that there are contradictory findings, but that in many services a clear bias is operating in that lower status clients tend to be assigned to lower status staff (Hsin et al , 1980). Other authors (e.g. Kline, 1973) suggest that staff may be "easing" such clients out of care.

Barriers to access

The CMHC movement in the USA hoped to overcome unnecessary barriers to care by removing the bureaucratic and cumbersome procedures often encountered by those in need of mental health care (Bratcher 1977). Some of the barriers which they hoped to remove were identified by Koltuv et al (1978) who found 48% of clients reported problems. These included inconvenient appointment times, therapists cancelling sessions, and unpleasant personnel on reception desks. Other features frequently noted in client complaints were problems encountered in trying to secure appointments and transport difficulties (Justice 1978, Kirchner 1981).

Emergency telephone services

A number of studies report on the inaccessibility of help by phone (Koltuv et al 1978). A survey of 99 CMHC's out of hours emergency telephone services conducted in 1977 (Wolfe, 1977), showed that 33% of the centres failed to answer the phones. The authors also note that concentrated effort was required to locate the emergency telephone numbers.

Self referrals

CMHC's appear to have facilitated self referral to some extent, in comparison to other sources of care such as public mental hospital, private mental hospital, and general hospital. The percentage of self referrals (those not dependent on the action of a professional), in relation to all referrals to a service, was highest in the Centres. (37% in CMHC's and 21% in private care; Ozarin 1974).

The problem of inappropriate usage and abuse of services thought to be engendered by the acceptance of self referrals, does not appear to be substantiated. Very few self referrals are judged to be unnecessary (Haw 1987, Hutton 1985). Some studies indicate that open access enables males to make more use of services This is found both in the UK (Hutton 1985, Haw 1987) and the USA.

Waiting times

The length of time a client is expected to wait for care is clearly an important feature of care from the clients' point of view. Long waiting times are a common complaint (Koltuv et al 1978), and a mailed survey of all users of one CMHC showed they valued minimal delay in receiving attention (Farber, 1975). There is some suggestion that outcomes are improved for clients seen immediately. In the UK one study showed that patients attending a mental health advice centre who were seen immediately showed more rapid improvement and satisfaction with services in comparison to those who were made to wait in an out patient clinic (Boardman, 1986).

There is some evidence to indicate that patients waiting times for care were reduced in some CMHCs (Beigel 1979) but complaints continued to be reported from others (Justice 1978, Kirchner 1981).

Temporal accessibility

Limited opening times is a feature of clients' reported dissatisfaction with services (Justice 1978). A survey by Bass (1970) showed that a majority of out patient units (71%) were only open in the day time, on five days a week. Few were open on evenings or weekends. Bouras (1982) reports that both professional care staff and the crisis intervention team in a UK advice centre, are only available during the day.

There is some evidence to indicate that there is a need for out of hours care. Haw (1987) studied the utilisation profile of an emergency clinic in the UK and found it to be heavily used out of hours, by self referred clients, especially those outside the catchment area. In a study in the US (Fiester et al 1975), non residents were presenting at emergency rooms with more serious problems than residents who were seen during regular working hours. In another study of out of hours demand, Blaney (1987) examines the source of referral for 212 clients coming to a general hospital psychiatric unit; the largest percentage were self referrals, 57%, general practitioners had referred 26% and the remaining 17% were from other community agencies. A large number of all these referrals were already in psychiatric care at other facilities.

Cognitive accessibility

Community awareness and 'visibility'

If a service is available this does not automatically guarantee that the community is aware of its existence. Access also depends upon knowledge of what is on offer, the acceptability of what is on offer, as well as how to make use of the service. There are a limited number studies of these aspects of accessibility. The studies summarised by Dowell & Ciarlo (1983) show the complexity of the matter. They found that approximately 17% of the residents of several catchment areas spontaneously named the CMHC when asked if they knew the service existed. This did not mean that they also knew where it was sited, how to go about using the service (procedural know how) or that they would select it as the place to go for their mental health problems. Only 8% of the residents in these studies knew its' location, and only 3% selected the CMHC as the place to go for help with mental health problems.

France et al (1978) studied all those seeking help with their mental health problems at a health service setting, and found that few, (3%) named the centre as a first resource for help, half of those referred by their physician to the centre did not go, and clients felt that the centre was a satellite of the state mental hospital, and were alarmed at the prospect of hospitalisation.

Greenblatt (1982) and Heinemann (1974) review studies which show poor community awareness in terms of both adequate information and understanding of how to make use of a CMHC. Heinemann (1974) notes that in one study, not one respondent named the centre as a place to turn to for psychiatric help, whilst 75% cited the city's general hospital located in another area. Even those living within a half mile radius of satellite clinics showed little awareness of their existence, or understanding of their role (between 40% and 90% of respondents in the areas studied did not know of them). For emergency care on weekends, the respondents were more likely to suggest the police than the CMHC.

Johnson (1975) reports on a community survey of two areas, one with and the other without a centre. They found differences in the way in which mental health needs were viewed in the two areas, and an indication that those served by a centre, were more likely to regard the mental health needs of their community as being adequately met. The response rates on which the findings rest were very low 10% in one area and 16% in the other.

Community gatekeepers e.g. clergy also displayed a lack of awareness of their CMHC. Scott et al (1984) found the levels of awareness among community gatekeepers to be higher than that for the community as a whole (53% and 37% respectively). Leaf et al (1985) studied the process of help seeking in a community interview survey of 4,838 residents (87% were white people, highly educated and high incomes). 51% of the respondents indicated a positive attitude towards the use of mental health services, whilst 83% mentioned barriers to care, which included lack of procedural know how, potential costs and time wasting. 24% felt their family may be upset by the stigmatising aspects of care, 53% felt their family doctor could probably help, and 29% suggested that the clergy might. The factors which were correlated with help seeking, were not the same as those related to frequency of contacts. The authors conclude that a lack of awareness of psychiatric matters and low receptivity to professional sources of help exerted the greatest barriers to obtaining care.

Publicity

Brounstein et al (1975) examined the brochures produced by 16 centres, and found them to be highly unsuitable for many target groups of clients, in that 9 out of 16 of them were judged to require at least a high school education to be understood. A content analysis of the mental health messages contained within pamphlets found that 60% of the messages were predominantly middle class, in ways that were often quite contrary to target clients' views. Morrison (1977) reports the results of a street survey by one centre to monitor visibility both before and after newspaper publicity. There was a significant increase in the number of people who were aware of the centre (from 28% to 53%).

Psychological accessibility (acceptability)

There are two main ways of looking at acceptability. One is to regard utilisation rates as indicators of the acceptability of services. A high take up rate and a low drop out rate could be regarded as indicators of the acceptability of the service. Dissatisfaction with service is unlikely to be expressed directly, and cannot be expressed by 'voting with one's feet' if there are no alternative services available.

Another indicator of acceptability can be obtained by conducting client satisfaction studies. These are not without their methodological problems. Consumer or client satisfaction with CMHC services is discussed in the chapter on service accountability.

Stigma

A major factor in the acceptability of services is the extent to which the service is seen as on which produces a 'spoiled social identity' for the service users. Insofar as the service does have this effect, it can be said to be stigmatising. One assumes that the greater the stigmatising effect of a service the less it will be used, or the more apprehensive people will be about using it. As far as we know, there are no studies of the stigmatising effect of CMHCs compared to other types of service. It is a major problem facing community based services which seek to be more accessible to all those in need of mental health care. However, there do not appear to be any clear solutions to the problem.

Specific ways of dealing with stigma of benefit to the client include the successful concealment of past history ("information management"; Jones, 1984), and the development of effective social skills, lost during institutionalisation, or underdeveloped in social situations ("tension management"; Jones,1984).

The consistent findings in studies of public attitudes towards mental patients are that those with mental health problems are thought to be dangerous, unreliable, best sent to hospital, often require readmissions, and are generally feared. Mental health facilities are typically regarded as noxious places (Maclean 1968, Dawe 1981, Dear 1982, Rosenberg and Atkinson 1977). Attempts to reduce the stigmatising effect of identifiable mental health facilities have involved the provision of service from disguised settings. These include the use of 'normal housing' and the use of 'store fronts'. Karno & Schwartz (1974) point out that professionals assume that such settings will be less alienating, less frightening and more familiar to low income groups. Two studies which specifically looked at the effects on uptake of store front services found there to be no major changes in the desired directions (Kinsey 1978, and Hedley et al, 1978). In the latter study, although there was an increase in the number of referrals (41%), there was no change in the nature of the population being served, except that more persons with no previous psychiatric history were attracted.

Consultation and education

The intention of the CMHC movement to include consultation and education services constituted an attempt to reduce the fear and misunderstanding surrounding mental health matters, and therefore was an indirect attempt to deal with the effects of stigma upon access. There is no study however which clearly demonstrates ways in which these barriers can be removed through educational means.

Reviewers of the movement in the USA have concluded that the issue of stigma was never adequately addressed, especially with regard to the deinstitutionalised patient (Bachrach 1983). CMHC's made very limited efforts in terms of consultation and education of the wider society; Cibulka (1981), found little emphasis on this aspect of work. When central funding was stopped, most centres ceased any activities of this kind altogether and the priority became earning income for the centre from reimburseable direct care services.

It would be inaccurate to assume that the US movement was incapable of reducing the stigma of mental health matters, as major efforts in this respect were not undertaken to any great extent, despite the wishes of centre staff. Stigma reduction is nevertheless still seen as a long term goal dependent on education of the wider society (Amesbury 1983, Okin 1978). This is perhaps an example of the triumph of hope over experience.

Acceptability to minority groups

We have already seen that CMHC services, although targeted at priority groups, did not attain nationwide coverage, and varied enormously in the extent to which they were used by minority groups. Of particular relevance are the findings that ethnic minorities failed to make use of services once referred to them. The failure to show up for the first appointment, the reluctance to attend for more than one appointment, and the early drop out from treatment could all be indicators of an unacceptable service. The selective use of certain forms of treatment for lower socioeconomic groups and the selection of other forms for higher groups might result in dissatisfaction among some service users.

There are other possible explanations for these findings. For instance, the rate of hospitalisation may be higher in respect of lower status groups because of the association between severity of disorder and lower status. This association arises (in part) because of social drift - the more severe disorder is responsible for the individual's decline in social status - so it is to be expected that lower groups have higher admission rates and may be overrepresented in hospital admissions. In the study by Greenblatt (1982), underusage of services was marked for all groups other than white people, and was related to their lack of knowledge of mental health services, mistrust of services and shame associated with mental problems. This was most marked for Hispanic groups. Greenblatt advocates active outreach, collaboration with communities, and the use of "indigenous professionals", in order to overcome these problems.

Ryan (1980), among others (e.g. Giordano 1976, Gary 1985), documents the communication problems between professionals and minority group clients. Essentially the same problems can be identified in the UK, and it is thought special efforts will be necessary to overcome the pervasive racism found in psychiatric service provision, (Littlewood 1986). This author documents the perpetuation of stereotyped notions about ethnic minorities among staff, the high levels of unmet need, the imbalances in numbers of staff from such groups and the continuing high rates of involuntary commitment.

Windle (1979) surveyed the efforts on the part of federally funded centres to encourage uptake by minority groups and compared these to their subsequent utilisation rates. Despite numerous documented efforts including; increasing the number of staff from ethnic minorities, increasing the number of satellite clinics in appropriate areas, increasing specific outreach efforts, providing transport, contacting clergy serving minority clients, holding workshops on minority issues, advertising in the Black peoples' media, there was no evidence of any improvement over one year.

Gary (1987) studied the attitudes of 411 black adults towards CMHCs. Fewer than 20% had negative attitudes, but 47% had neutral attitudes. Female gender, married status and a high level of racial consciousness were associated with more positive attitudes.

Drop outs and 'no shows'

An important indicator of the acceptability of care to clients referred to community mental health services is the extent to which they vote with their feet. 'No shows', are those people who do not turn up for their initial appointment,(rates vary between 57% and 37%) and drop outs, are those who do not complete the course of care offered to them (range between 20% and 50%).

Estimates of the proportions of clients who drop out of care are reviewed by Dowell & Ciarlo (1983). In 1974 NIMH data showed that over 35% of 'discontinued' clients were not referred to another treatment resource. For 90% of these cases the reasons given for nonreferral was dropping out of treatment. In a study of one centre in Spanish Harlem in New York, Rosen et al

(1980) report that 16% failed to return for their second appointment, and later 8% left treatment after two visits. The initial
drop outs were significantly more likely to be black clients.
Giordano (1976), among others, sees the failure to understand
the cultural diversity of clients, as the main reason for centres
inability to keep clients in care.

An initial reluctance to come to services is common in ethnic
minority groups. They form a significant percentage of those who
do not turn up for initial appointments (Kluger 1983; Allan,
1988). Kluger found that indication that the number of no shows
was reduced by the use of prompts, reminders and 'orientation'
to services. The latter included, an explanation as to how services
worked, the amounts of money which would be involved, what to
expect on admission to the Centre, and a display of interest on
the part of the staff in the clients welfare. The instigation of the
orientation effort, reduced the number of no shows from 37% to
23%.

It seems that at least some of the problems of accessibility for
this group, were to do with their lack of procedural know how in
relation to provision, and their anticipation of a poor response
from staff, both of which were ameliorated to some extent by the
orientation program. Attempts to account for the low acceptability of care for minority groups, have drawn attention to the
communication problems thought to exist between members of
different cultural and status groups. These lead to poor understanding of clients' perspectives by staff. Evidence of conflict in
interests between clients and therapists is plentiful (Dinkel et al
1981; Windle et al 1981; Sullivan 1981; Love 1979; Freed et al,
1972; Zisook, 1978).

Some success has been reported in the use of cultural training
orientation for staff. This has been shown to increase the reported satisfaction of clients after the staff training (Yamanoto
1984). The use of indigenous paraprofessionals is also found to
increase the relevance and acceptability of care offered (Ozarin
1975), especially in the case of the use of a service guide, whose
presence and subsequent absence markedly affected uptake of
services (Raft et al 1976) (see Chapter 2).

Another study confirms that better informed clients are more
receptive to services offered. Otto (1974), found that client expectations of care were directly related to subsequent uptake and
participation (drop outs tended to have high expectations on
admission to care and were disappointed when programs did not
match up) , and that preparation of clients especially providing
accurate information about the service improves utilisation. The
use of a community liaison worker helped to substantially reduce
the number of no shows among ex hospital patients (Krebs 1971).

Zisook (1978) studied drop outs in an out patient clinic and
found that they did not feel they had been understood by staff,
and that they were dissatisfied with the initial session offered to

them. Girard (1979) interviewed equal numbers of those who came for their first appointment and those who did not, and found that the difference lay in the latter's feeling that their needs had not been appropriately addressed. Larsen (1979) found there to be a direct relationship between no shows, and long delays between initial contact and appointments. Richer (1979) and others (Love, 1979; Leaf et al 1985) found clients dropped out because of the cost of care and the length of waiting lists. Similar results have been reported by Callister & Berger (1980) who identified cost, waiting period and transportation problems among the main reasons for drop-out.

Pekarik (1983) traced 45% of treatment drop outs and found the following were the main reasons. 39% felt they had no need for the service, 20% found the care on offer inconvenient to obtain (transport, hours, money, and time), 17% disliked the services, 9% went elsewhere for care, and the remainder dropped out for a variety of reasons, such as moving out of the area, or the program ceased. The drop outs were also given a self report brief symptom inventory to complete on admission and follow up, which showed that only the group claiming to be dissatisfied with the services reported no change in the prevalence of symptoms. Both those who found the services cumbersome to use, and those who claimed to have no further need for services, showed significant improvement in symptom severity.

The authors conclude that the study shows that treatment drop outs are not an homogeneous group of treatment failures, in that they may contain numbers of those who have improved sufficiently to warrant cessation of treatment (at least in their own view). In terms of the acceptability of services, however it is important to note that at least a quarter of treatment drop outs find the service unacceptable.

Summary and conclusions

1

As one of the main goals of the CMHC movement in the USA, accessibility has received a good deal of attention. It is a multifaceted concept which requires clarification (Holland, 1975). A major problem is the way in which several different concepts are nested within one global concept of accessibility.

2

We located the following meanings of accessibility and acceptability in the literature: geographic accessibility, or **proximity**; **cognitive** (do people know where the service is, what it is for, who is eligible, and how to access it?); **bureaucratic** (is there a referral system, is there a waiting list etc.?) and **psychological**. The last of these is synonymous with **acceptability** (is it the sort of service which the person wants, likes and is satisfied with?).

3

Many service delivery strategies were used in an attempt to improve access to services; firm evidence for their efficacy is hard to find.

4

CMHCs partially achieved one of their major objectives, in that services were brought to some areas where previously there had been none (Ozarin 1971). The CMHC mandate improved coverage but it was not until later that the de facto mental health service (the extent to which family physicians dealt with mental health problems) was revealed (Regier et al, 1978). In this important respect the USA and the UK are remarkably similar.

5

There are several reasons why a simple judgment about the accessibility of CMHC services cannot be made. The main one is the great variability between centres. The proportion of the service used by known priority groups varies from none, in some cases, to all, in others. Rothman and Kay (1982), document this massive variability across centres. In terms of serving the poor the range across centres was from 10% to 96% of centre case loads; for schizophrenia the range was from 0% to 100%; for alcoholism from 0% to 47% ; for non-psychotic disorders, 0% to 67%; and for no mental disturbance from 0% to 98%.

6

Geographic accessibility: Brandon (1975) found that social characteristics of clients were the main determinants of uptake, regardless of the siting of services. Some clients will travel to utilise services regardless of where they are provided, whilst others will ignore the services even if they are nearby. In fact, the degree of conviction that providing services locally improves access would appear to be inversely related to the amount of evidence that it does so.

7

Bureaucratic accessibility: The CMHC movement hoped to overcome unnecessary barriers to care by removing the bureaucratic and cumbersome procedures often encountered by those in need of mental health care. Some of the barriers which they hoped to remove were identified by Koltuv et al (1978). These included inconvenient appointment times, therapists cancelling sessions, and unpleasant personnel on reception desks, problems encountered in trying to secure appointments and transport difficulties (Justice 1978, Kirchner 1981). CMHC's appear to have facilitated self referral to some extent, in comparison to other sources of care such as public mental hospital, private mental hospital, and general hospital. The problem of inappropriate usage and abuse of services thought to be engendered by the acceptance of self referrals, does not appear to be substantiated. Very few self referrals are judged to be unnecessary (Haw 1987, Hutton 1985). Some studies indicate that open access enables males to make more use of services This is found both in the UK (Hutton 1985, Haw 1987) and the USA.

8

Cognitive accessibility: Community awareness and 'visibility'- if a service is available this does not automatically guarantee that the community is aware of its existence. Access also depends upon knowledge of what is on offer, the acceptability of what is on offer, as well as how to make use of the service. Dowell & Ciarlo (1983) found that approximately 17% of the residents of several catchment areas spontaneously named the CMHC when asked if they knew the service existed. This did not mean that they also knew where it was sited, how to go about using the service (procedural know how) or that they would select it as the place to go for their mental health problems. Only 8% of the residents in these studies knew its' location, and only 3% selected the CMHC as the place to go for help with mental health problems.

9

Psychological accessibility (Acceptability): As far as we know, there are no studies of the stigmatising effect of CMHCs compared to other types of service. Stigma is a major problem facing community based services which seek to be more accessible to all those in need of mental health care. However, there do not appear to be any easy solutions to the problem (Jones,1984).

10

Ethnic minorities failed to make use of services once referred to them. The failure to show up for the first appointment, the reluctance to attend for more than one appointment, and the early drop out form treatment could all be indicators of an unacceptable service. In a study by Greenblatt (1982), underusage of services was marked for all groups other than white people, and was related to their lack of knowledge of mental health services,

mistrust of services and shame associated with mental problems.
11
'No shows' do not turn up for their initial appointment,(rates vary between 57% and 37%) and drop outs do not complete the course of care offered to them (range between 20% and 50%). Kluger (1983) found that the number of no shows could be reduced by the use of prompts, reminders and 'orientation' to services. The latter included, an explanation as to how services worked, the amounts of money which would be involved, what to expect on admission to the Centre, and a display of interest on the part of the staff in the clients welfare. The instigation of the orientation effort, reduced the number of no shows from 37% to 23%.

References

Abrams, P. (1977). Community Care: Some Research Problems and Priorities. *Policy and Politics* 6:125-151.

Allan, A.T. (1988) No-shows at a Community Mental Health Clinic: a Pilot Study. *Int.J.Soc.Psychiat.* 34(1):40-46.

Amesbury, W.H. (1983) The comprehensive mental health system. *Perspectives in Psychiatric Care* 21(1):31-33.

Armstrong, H.E. et al (1984). Service Utilization by black & white clients in urban CMHC. *C.M.H. Journal* 20(4):269-81.

Bachrach,L. (1984). Asylum and chronically ill psychiatric patients. *Am.J.Psychiat.* 141(8):975-978.

Bachrach, L.L. (1983). Deinstitutionalisation. *Hospital and Community Psychiatry*, 34(2).

Bass,R. (1970). *The accessibility of C.M.H.C.* NIMH, Maryland.

Beigel, A. (1979). Evaluation on a Shoe-string. In Hargreaves, et al (1979) *op. cit.*

Blaney, D. and West, A. (1987). Out of Hours referrals to a general psychiatric hospital. *Health Bulletin* 45:67-70.

Boardman, A.P. et al (1986). Evaluation of a CMHC. *Acta Psych.Belg.* :402-406.

Borus, J.F. (1978). Issues Critical to Survival of C.M.H. *American Journal of Psychiatry* 135(9):1029-1035.

Bouras, N. (1982). Development of the mental health advice centre in Lewisham Health District. *Health Trends* 14(3):65-68.

Bratcher, M. (1977). The CMHC: An Effective Approach to M.H. Care *J. of Tennessee Medical Association* 70(4):259-260.

Brounstein, D.A. et al (1975). Readability of CMHC brochures for client consumption. *J.Comm Psych.* 3(2):193-195.

Brown, P. (1984). *Transfer of Care.* RKP, London.

Callister, s. & Berger, M. (1980) *A Study of Failures of Follow-Through for Initial Mental Health Interviews.* Paper presented to the Annual Convention of the Rocky Mountain Psychologi cal Association, Tucson, Arizona.

Cibulka, J.G. (1981). Special Investigation - Citizen participation C.M.H. Services. *C.M.H. Journal* 17(1):19.

Cob, C.W. (1972). CMH Services & the lower socio-economic classes *Am.J.Orthopsych.* 42(3):404-14.

Dawe, A.M. (1981). Value for money. *Nursing Mirror* July 29.

Dear, M.J. & Taylor, S.M. (1982). *Not on our street.* Pion Ltd. London.

Derisi, W. et al. (1983). Impact of deinstitutionalisation on the California State hospital population. *Hosp. & Comm. Psych.* 34(2):140-44.

Dinkel, et al (1981). Citizen Participation in C.M.H.C. Program Evaluation-Neglected Potential. *Comm. M.H. Journal* 17:54-65.

Dowell, D.A. & Ciarlo, J.A. (1983). Overview of the C.M.H.C. Program from an Evaluation Perspective. *Comm.M.H.Journal.* 19:95-125.

Du Sautoy,T.(1987). A Parting Shot. *Community Care* 26 Feb: 23-25.

Farber, D.A. (1975). Study of clients reactions to initial contacts with a CMHC. *Smith College Studies in Social Work* 46(1):44-5.

Fiester, A.R., Silverman, W.H. & Beech, R.P. (1975). Problems involved in delivering emergency services in hospital based CMHCs *J.Comm.Psychol.* 3(2):188-192.

France, R.D. et al (1978). Referral of patients from primary care physicians. *J. Nerv.Mental Dis.* 166:594-598.

Freed, H.M. et al (1972). Community mental health second class treatment. *Mental Hygiene* 56(3):256-9.

Gary, L.E. (1985).Attitudes towards human service organisation-*J.App.Behav.Sci.* 21(4):445-458.

Gary, L.E. (1987) Attitudes of Black Adults Toward Community Mental Health Centres. *Hosp.Comm.Psychiat.* 38(10):1100-1105.

Giordano, A. (1976). Community Mental Health in a Pluralistic Society. *Int.J.Ment.Health* 5(2):5-15.

Girard, D.P. (1979). A Study of pre-take drop-out of South Shore CMHC. *Dissertation Abs. Int.* 40(5):2362-B Ann Arbor, Mich.

Goodman, A.B. (1979). Ethnic and class factors affecting mental health clinic services. *Eval. & prog.Planning* 2:159-71.

Gorman, M (1976). Community Absorption of the Mentally Ill. *Comm.M.H. Journal* 12(2):347-55.

Greenblatt, M. & Beceira, R. (1982). *Social Networks & Mental Health: An Overview.*

Hagedorn, H.J. et al (1976) *A Working Manual of Simple Program Evaluation Techniques for CMHCs.* NIMH DHEW Publication No.(ADM) 76-404.

Hall, G.B. (1988) Monitoring and Predicting Community Mental Centre Utilization in Aukland,NewZealand.*Soc.Sci.Med.* 26(1):55-70.

Hart, N.T. (1972). Delivery of services to lower socio-economic groups. *Am.J.Psych* 129.

Haw, C. (1987). Patients at a psychiatric walk in clinic In *Bulletin of the R.C. Psych.*

Hedley, R.A. et al (1970). Community mental health teams *Soc.Sci. & Med* 12(4):265-270.

Heinemann, S.H. (1974). The C.M.H.C. and community awareness. *Comm.M.H.Journal* 10(2):221-227.

Holland, B.C. (1975). Evaluation of criticisms of the community mental health movement. In Barton & Sanborn, Assessment of the Community Mental Health Movement, *op.cit.*

Hsin, W. et al (1980). Ethnic specificity in relative minority use and staff. *Comm.M.H.Journ.* 16(2).

Hutton, F. (1985). Self Referrals to a C.M.H.C.- A Three Year Study. *Brit. J. Psych.* 147:540-544.

Johnson, J.J. (1975). CMHC Evaluation: A Survey of mental health problems and professional services. *Evaluation* 2(2):18.

Jones, K. & Poleti, A. (1984). Transformation of the asylum: The Italian Experience. *Int. J. Mental Health*

Justice, B. et al (1978). A Client satisfaction survey of one element in evaluation. *Comm.M.H.Journal* 14(3):248-252.

Karno, M. & Schwartz, D.A. (1974). *C.M.H. Reflections and exploration.* Spectrum, New York.

Kirchner, J.H. (1981). Patient feedback on satisfaction with direct services received at a CMHC. *Psychotherapy* 18(3):359-64.

Kline, J. et al (1973). Treatment Dropouts from a CMHC.*Comm.M.H. Journal* 9(4):354.

Kluger, M.P. (1983). Strategies for reducing initial appointments in a CMHC. *Comm.M.H.Journal* 19(2):137.

Koltuv, M. Basheeruddin, A. & Meyer, M. (1978). A Study of outpatient satisfaction with mental health centre services *Hosp. & Comm. Psychiat.* 29(3).

Krebs, R. (1977). Using attendance as a means of evaluating CMHC progress. *Comm.M.H. Journal* 7:1.

Lang, C.L. (1981). Good cases - bad cases, client selection in a CMHC. *Urban Life* 10:289-309.

Larsen, D.L. (1979). Assessment of client/patient satisfaction *Eval. & Program Planning* 2:197-207.

Leaf, P.J. et al. (1985) Contact with health professionals for treatment of psychiatric problems. *Med. Care* 23(12):1322-37.

Levin,G. Wilder, J.F. & Gilbert, J. (1978). Identifying and meeting client's needs in six CMHCs. *Hosp. & Comm. Psychiat.* 29(3).

Littlewood, R. (1986). Psychiatric Services for Black and other minority groups in Birmingham. Workshop Paper *op.cit.*

Love, R.E. et al (1979). The user satisfaction survey. *Eval. & The Health Professionals* 1(5):42-54.

Macintyre, S. (1986). Patterning of health by social position in contemporary Britain. *Soc. Sci. & Med.* 23(4):339-415.

Maclean, U (1986). 1966 Edinburgh survey of community attitudes to mental illness. *Health Bulletin* XXVI (3):23-57.

Mollica, R.F. et al (1980). Equity and Psychiatric Care of Black Patients. *J.Nerv.Ment.Dis.* 168(5):279-86.

Morrison, J.K. et al (1977). Effect of newspaper publicity on a C.M.H.C. *Comm.M.H.Journal* 13(1):58-61.

N.I.M.H. (1980). *News & Notes* :70-77.

NIMH (1973). *Impact of evaluation methodology.* Publication No. 250744, Springfield, VA.

Okin, R.L. (1978). Future of State Mental Health Programs for Chronic Psychiatric Patient in the Community. *Am Psych. Assoc.* 135(11):1355-1358.

Orden, S.R. & Sticking, C.B. (1971) *Relationships between community mental health centres and other caregiving agencies.* Springfield, VA.

Otto, J. & Moos, R. (1974). Patient expectations and attendance in community treatment programs. *Comm.M.H. Journal* 10(1).

Ozarin, L. (1971). Experience with CMHCs. *Am.J. Psychiat.* 127(7):912.

Ozarin, L. (1974). Psychiatric inpatients: who, where, and future *Am.J.Psychiat.* 131(1):98-101.

Ozarin, L.D. (1975). C.M.H. does it work : review of the literature. In Barton & Sandborn, *op. cit.*

Pardes, H. & Stockdill, J.W. (1983). Overview of the CMHC program from an evaluation perspective. *Comm.M.H. Journal* 19(2)126-8.

Pekarik, G. (1983). Improvement in clients - reasons for dropping out. *J.Clin.Psychol.* 39(6):910-13.

Phillips, P.B. (1976). CMHCs - Or is there a better way? *J.Florida Med. Asn* 63(5):353.

Phillips, P.B. (1981) CMHCs - Pros & Cons. *J.Florida Med. Asn.* Feb 103-107.

Raft, D.D. et al (1976). Using a service guide to provide comprehensive care in a rural CMHC. *Hosp. & Comm. Psych.* 27(8):553-9.

Richer, A. (1979) Factors associated with continuance and non-continuance in out-patient psychotherapy at a CMHC: The client's perspective. *Dissertation Abstracts International.* Ann Arbor, Michigan.

Rosen, A. et al (1980). Utilization patterns of a CMHC in an urban ghetto. *Hosp. & Comm Psych.* 31:702-704.

Rosenberg, G & Atkinson, L. (1977). Attitudes towards mental illness in the working class. *Soc.Wk. in Health Care* 3(1):77-86.

Rothman, J & Kay, T. (1982). CMHCs and Family Service Agencies *Soc. Wk. Research & Abstracts* 10-16.

Rumer, R. (1978). CMHCs - Politics to therapy. *J. Health Politics, Policy & Law* 2(4):531-559.

Ryan, R.A. (1980). A Community Perspective for mental health research. *Social Casework*

Scott, R.R. et al (1984). Assessing a CMHC's impact & awareness of services. *J.Comm.Psychol.* 12(1):61-66.

Shepherd, M. (1987). Mental Illness and primary care. *Am.J.Pub. Health* 12-13.

Siegel, R. (1973) Mental health volunteers as change agents. *Am.J.Comm.Psych.* 1:138-158.

Springer, S.M. (1977). Social Class and Psychiatric treatment of adults in the mental hospital. *J.Health & Soc.Behav.* 18:317-325.

Sullivan, J.M. et al (1981). Monitoring frequency of clients problems. *Evaluation Review* 5(6):822-833.

Townsend, P. & Davidson, N. (1982). *Inequalities in Health.* Penguin Books, London.

Walker, A. (1988) Tendering Care. *New Society*, 22 Jan.18-19.

White, S. (1987). What should an ideal emergency psychiatry service be like. *Bulletin of the Royal College of Psychiatrists* 11:326-9.

Windle, C. (1979). Stimulating the equality of CMHC services to non whites. *Comm.M.H. Journal* 15(2):155-62.

Windle, C., Bass, R.D. & Gray, L. (1987) The impact of federally funded CMHCs on local mental health service systems. *Hosp. Comm. Psychiat.* 38(7):729-734.

Windle, C., Poppen, P.J., Thompson, J.W. & Marvelle, K. (1988a) Types of Patients Served by Various Providers of Outpatient Care in CMHCs. *Am.J.Psychiat.* 145(4):457-463.

Windle, C., Thompson, J.W., Goldman, H.H. & Naierman, N. (1988b) Treatment of Patients with No Diagnosable Mental Disorders in CMHCs. *Hosp.Comm.Psychiat.* 39(7):753-758.

Yamanoto, J. (1984). Orienting therapists' and patients' needs to increase patient satisfaction. *Am.J.Psychiat.* 141(2):274.

Zisook, S. et al (1978). Out patient requests, initial sessions and attendance. *Int. J. Psychiat.in.Med.* 9:339-350.

4 Efficient services

Introduction

The concept of efficiency is most frequently applied to the delivery of mental health services through the use of cost-benefit or cost effectiveness analyses. A number of authors review the use of cost-benefit analysis and similar methods in the assessment of the efficiency of mental health services, in particular community mental health centers. These include Bootman, 1979; Dowell and Ciarlo, 1983 ; Frank, 1981;, Glass and Goldberg,1977; Keisler 1985; Levin, 1975; May 1970,1971; Rothenberg 1975; and Sharfstein and Clark 1978. One or two articles provide useful conceptual summaries. Others report the use of these analyses in practice. Some are based on small numbers, others are methodologically inadequate. A number relate to community alternatives to mental hospitals rather than to CMHCs specifically.

In this section of the review we will examine the conceptual issues, cost-benefit and cost-effectiveness studies of CMHCs and alternatives to mental hospital treatment, the efficiency of CMHCs in terms of target efficiency (see below) and recent papers on the impact of economic stringency on CMHCs. In terms of the framework applied in this book all these studies concern identified psychiatric patients. There has been some debate about the costs of treating hidden psychiatric morbidity and this is briefly reported below. The economic results of efforts to prevent mental health problems can only be surmised as no adequate cost-benefit studies could be located.

Conceptual framework

The most useful conceptual frameworks are given by Levin (1975) and Bootman (1979). A similar framework, unrelated to CMHCs is given by Martin Knapp (1984).

Cost-benefit analysis compares the monetary value of benefits with the monetary value of costs. This enables comparison of rates of return on investment, net differences between costs and benefits, and benefit to cost ratios. A crucial assumption for conducting cost-benefit analyses is that the benefits or outcomes can be given a monetary value. This is often not possible in psychosocial treatment programmes.

In these circumstances a **cost-effectiveness** approach, where the impact of the programme is assessed in non-monetary terms, may be more suitable. A cost-benefit approach can sometimes be added on to a cost effectiveness study, if physical or psychological outcomes can be converted into monetary values.

Cost-utility analysis relies more heavily on qualitative factors, such as subjective judgements, than do either of the other two methods. There are two ways in which subjective judgements may be included. First, by including the personal views of the decision makers - concerning the relative value to them of the alternative outcomes (Fisher, 1964). Second, by including the personal views of the service recipients - concerning improvements in their circumstances (Knapp, 1984). In the latter, the assessment of changes in the client's perceived quality of life has attracted increased attention in recent years, particularly in the field of health care outcomes (Flanagan, 1982; Levine, 1987).

Common to each of these approaches is the need to measure **costs**. A frequent failing in estimating costs is the use of a narrow definition, particularly one which only includes accounting costs or direct expenditures. This phenomenon has been observed on both sides of the Atlantic (Levin, 1975; Williams, 1977). The term 'costs' should be used to refer to the value of all the resources associated with any particular action. The expenditure of resources in one way precludes its use in another and this concept of sacrifice, or 'opportunity cost' should be included in the measurement of costs. Williams (1977) is of the opinion that our preoccupation with cash-based, input-oriented budgetary systems (or 'cash-consciousness') is a 'major obstacle to greater efficiency', and that this will not change 'until the economist's notion of opportunity cost (in real resource terms) becomes dominant in everyone's thinking'.

Further problems caused by the narrow definition of costs include: the failure to include the cost of client time in attending for treatment and the failure to include the costs borne by other 'constituencies', such as family, or other sectors of welfare, such as housing providers.

Measuring costs presents further difficulties. In both the USA and the UK the collection of cost data has been infrequent in evaluation studies. It has rarely been included as part of the routine data collection of projects. Even when data are produced as part of an experimental programme, it is by no means certain that this information can be used as the basis for large scale policy planning and development. Levin (1975) advocates an 'ingredients approach' (listing the ingredients, or inputs, and assigning costs to them). He suggests that the items which consume most of the programme budget should receive most of one's attention when estimating costs. A category that accounts for no more than 5% of the budget should not receive more than 5% of one's time!

Measuring costs and benefits takes place over time, and we may therefore become involved in comparing costs and benefits at times when the value of money is different. In addition, by investing money now, on a mental health project, we not only forego the benefit of spending that money on an alternative project, but we also forego interest payments. The procedure for determining the present value of a cost in the future is known as **discounting** and the discounting of future values back to the present time is the reverse of compounding interest. Costs are converted into present values by using a **discount rate**. In the UK the Treasury recommends a particular numerical value for use in public sector cost-benefit analyses (Knapp, 1984).

If the major costs of the project are in the early years and the benefits mainly occur towards the end, a discount rate which is too high will tend to undervalue the present benefits relative to the costs. One which is too low will undervalue the costs relative to the benefits.

Finally when making cost comparisons between projects, in relation to cost-effectiveness for instance, the appropriate costs must be used. When the alternative programmes are of approximately equal effectiveness then the **total costs** may be compared. When programmes differ in terms of their effectiveness it is advisable to use **average cost** per unit of effectiveness. The outcomes of the programmes must be measured in the same effectiveness units. A drawback of this approach is that programmes with large fixed costs (such as those residential solutions which involve new building) will show high average costs for low levels of output.

In some cases it is the **marginal** cost that is the relevant measure. This is particularly true when the cost per unit of effectiveness changes according to the scale of the programme. The marginal cost is the cost of an additional unit of output. Marginal cost effectiveness comparisons are also used when decision makers must allocate budget increases or decreases between competing parts of a service.

Efficiency

None of the articles we have reviewed so far have been specifically concerned with efficiency. In order to look at the relevant literature from the point of view of efficiency we need a framework. The concepts of efficiency in Knapp (1984) provides us with such a framework.

Efficiency is achieved by allocating resources to generate the maximum possible output. Something is **technically efficient** when it produces a maximum set of outputs from a given amount of inputs. **Price efficiency** occurs when a given level of output is produced at minimum cost. **Target efficiency** is the efficiency with which resources are allocated to and among those for whom receipt has been judged the most cost effective method of intervention. There are two types of target efficiency, horizontal and vertical.

Horizontal target efficiency is the extent to which those deemed to be in need of a service actually receive it. **Vertical target efficiency** is the extent to which the available resources are used by those deemed to be in need.

A technically efficient service which is also price efficient can be called cost-effective, because it produces the given output at minimum cost. It is worth noting that simply minimising the costs of inputs, does not necessarily lead to increased efficiency. One has to be concerned about the nature and level of outputs, and the relationship between inputs and outputs. A service cannot be efficient if it not effective, but services will differ in the ration of their inputs to their outputs. This capacity to produce is known as **productivity**. Productivity measures which take account of all inputs, and all outputs are not very different from measures of technical efficiency. An interesting concept, known as **X-efficiency** (or sometimes X-inefficiency) occurs when an input, or combination of inputs, is not used effectively. The difference between the actual output and the maximum output attributable to that input, is a measure of the degree of X-efficiency. The most common way in which this phenomenon presents itself in mental health service delivery, is in connection with the mixture of treatments or of personnel providing care for individual patients. The most optimal combinations will be efficient, but since we know relatively little about the variation in the effectiveness of different combinations of treatment inputs, in the mental health field, it is almost certain that much of the care provided is X-inefficient. The only paper which we have been able to find which bears on this subject, (Frank & Taube,1987) is reviewed in detail below.

For the purposes of making an assessment of the efficiency of CMHCs the concepts of horizontal and vertical target efficiency are useful. One can assess the horizontal target efficiency of a CMHC by looking at the needs of the population to be served and comparing this with the utilization rates of groups of people who are deemed to be in need of the service. One can assess the vertical target efficiency of a CMHC by looking at the characteristics of users against the stated eligibility criteria for service provision or against stated target groups. One must keep in mind the fact that target efficiencies as defined here assume that the resources provided have been judged to be the most cost-effective available. As we shall see from the studies of cost effectiveness below, deciding what constitututes the most cost-effective service depends upon complicated calculations and judgements about costs and benefits. In general the literature is small and findings from one centre may be inapplicable in another. Results for long-term patients are certain to differ from those of acute patients.

We have been unable to locate any studies of cost-utility analysis although the Goldberg & Jones study reviewed below, perhaps comes closest to this in intention. The remainder of the literature can be divided into cost-benefit and cost-effectiveness studies, both of which have been conducted in CMHCs and in other settings, such as community services, or services providing an alternative to mental hospital. Target efficiency as such does not appear in the literature. However several papers give data which are relevant to the concepts of horizontal and vertical target efficiency, and these are reviewed. The chapter concludes with a brief examination of the impact of economic cutbacks on CMHCs.

Reviews of cost-effectiveness

There are a number of papers which review cost-effectiveness concepts and which discuss various aspects of efficiency (Hagedorn, 1976; May, 1970; Rothenberg, 1975). On the whole these papers do not refer to specific experiments. Bootman et al's (1979) review of cost-benefit analysis is the easiest to follow, and Frank's review (1981) contains the most up-to-date review of the literature. Keisler (1985) reviewed studies of modes of care used instead of hospitalization. He excluded all studies which did not meet the following criteria: all patients should be seriously disturbed; randomly assigned to conditions of treatment; treatment should be specified, and patient characteristics described; and patient progress tracked over time. He insisted on the random assignment criterion because random assignment avoids the problem of inadequate matching due to inadequate assessment and diagnosis, and the inability to be sufficiently precise about critical therapeutic agents.

Keisler found 10 such experiments. His overall conclusions were that ' for the vast majority of patients now being assigned to inpatient units in mental institutions, care of at least equal impact could be otherwise provided. There is not an instance..in which hospitalisation had any positive impact on the average patient which exceeded that of the alternative care investigated in the study'. Most significantly for the purpose of the present chapter he asserted that ' ..in no case did the cost of alternative care exceed that of inpatient care.' In some of the studies which he included, cost data was not provided and in others the cost data measurement was inadequate. The studies which included adequate cost data are reviewed, along with others, below.

Cost-benefit studies in CMHCs

On the basis of a single case-study, Sharfstein and Nafziser (1976) conclude that the case 'demonstrates that the benefits of community care far outweigh the costs in both dollars and human terms'. Their method and their measures do not justify this conclusion. They report the costs and benefits of caring for a discharged, middle-aged female patient. The costs of care in the community included professional support and treatment, interagency conference costs, backup medical care, and emergency visits to the CMHC. The benefits measured were the savings through the use of non-hospital services, increased economic output of the patient, and improved well-being of the patient (not quantified).

In the first year in the community the costs amounted to $2,100. By the third year the cost was $640. This compares well with the 'cost' (measurement unspecified) of the state hospital of $5,902, the day care programme in the CHMC, $5,809, and inpatient care in the CMHC, $15,476. She represents one of the more suitable cases for discharge to the community. She was able to work in the homemaker scheme, thereby reducing her dependence on both the support services and income maintenance services. Only a proportion of discharged patients can expect to function at this level, and those who cannot will cost more to support.

Halpern (1977) reports on the use of Output Value Analysis (OVA) at the Fort Logan Mental Health Center. This analyis is a form of cost-benefit analysis since it assumes that improvements in patient functioning - even at a subjective level - can be given dollar values.

The economic value of treatment output is measured on two dimensions - estimated economic productivity on the basis of earned income (in the year after discharge), and the economic value of the patients' response to treatment. This 'estimated response percentage' was calculated by constructing a matrix based on four levels of impairment at admission and five at discharge. The resulting 20 cells were assigned scores based on clinicians' and clinical administrators' judgements. After consulting insurance company paymemt levels, for physical injury, (the latter ranged from 25000 dollars to 50000 dollars) a single dollar value of 10000 was used to multiply the matrix scores, thereby arriving at the dollar-value of improvement.

The impairment measures used in this study reflect resource utilization - the anticipated resource utilisation score (Potter, Halpern and Binner, 1974). This is essentially a prediction, made at the time of admission, of the amount of resources a patient would require for treatment. It is based on the past costs of treating patients with similar demographic characteristics and mental state.

The results of the initial analysis showed that the Adult Psychiatry division was realizing an overall return of approximately $3.00 in benefits for each dollar of investment' (Binner ,Halpern and Potter 1972). Different teams in the Fort Logan adult psychiatric division varied in their returns on dollars invested, from a low of $2.35 to $4.50.

The use of cost measures based on the past costs of similar patients almost certainly makes the cost assessment highly inaccurate for any individual patient. The manner in which dollar values were assigned to patient improvement in this study is questionable. The size of the rate of return is highly dependent upon this figure (10000 dollars). However. so long as the assumptions remain constant, a comparison would be possible between, for example, output value indices of two different programs. A study of this sort would be less influenced by the probable inaccuracy of certain of the internal assumptions of the model.

In another study Binner et al (1973) used this form of analysis to show that short low-intensity programs gave the highest rate of return but long low intensity programmes yield the best level of response.

Cost-effectiveness studies in CMHCs

Luft L.L. and Fakhouri J. (1979) compared hospital day care and community day care at the Peninsula hospital community mental health centre in Burlingame, California. The study was not a comparison of the two forms of care versus one another, but an assessment of the extent to which each was able to reduce hospitalization, based on their use of services in the period prior to and after the patients first admission to the two day care programs. The major weakness of this investigation is that patients were not randomly assigned to the two forms of care, and so the results are influenced by the significant differences between the two groups.

Hospital day care included occupational therapy and group therapy, and aimed to increase socialization, independence and insight. Community day care was located in community centres, such as church halls, and aimed to provide structured social experiences, community involvement and leisure time planning. It aimed to decrease dependency on hospital care and provide support for functioning in the community. Both forms of day care accepted all diagnostic groups, but the community day care (CDC) patients were more likely to have a previous history of psychiatric treatment. The hospital day care group (HDC) were more likely to be suffering from an acute episode. HDC patients had to be able to benefit from insight oriented psychotherapy.

CDC was on offer twice a week for four hours a day. HDC was offered every day. 28 patients a day attended HDC and 20 attended CDC. Each CDC had two staff members, a mental health worker and a voluntary nurse, one on a permanent basis and one rotating between the CDCs.

Data were collected between June 1971 and June 1973 at the HDC,and between March 1971 and October 1975 at the CDCs. Of 371 first admissions 275 met the criterion of having had at least 5 days in treatment in a partial care program; 182 HDC, 47 CDC, and 46 in both. Patients who had been treated in both settings were dropped from the analysis. 49 (27%) patients in HDC had not had previous in-patient admissions, compared with 19 (40%) in the CDC setting. CDC patients were significantly older than those in HDC, more were male, more had prior admissions, and were more likely to be married and widowed. HDC patients were more likely to be single, divorced and separated.

The costs which were examined included - hospital charges; salaries; upkeep costs; depreciation; rent; liability insurance; dietary expenses; medical records, peer review and evaluation costs; and overheads. Benefits were defined as the difference between the costs of in-patient and emergency room use during the pre- and post-admission periods. Effectiveness is, therefore, defined in a particularly narrow way in this investigation.

Neither program showed a decrease in the use of the emergency room. In fact HDC patients showed increase on the average. The CDC benefit-cost ratio was 3.36, and 6.53 for those with prior hospitalisation. The HDC benefit-cost ratio was .55 overall and 1.02 for the prior hospitalisation group. The savings made per reduction in the number of in-patient days (comparing pre- and post-admission periods) was $236 for HDC and $38 for CDC.

These findings are direct result of the differences between the groups of patients studied. The HDC group had more patients with previous admissions. This would mean they were more difficult and more costly to treat, hence the low b-c ratio. Additionally there was much more scope to make savings because of their previous, more costly in-patient treatment. By contrast CDC patients were receiving low level, inexpensive and less frequent care in the community, making a high b-c ratio more easily achieved. Savings made by using CDC were bound to be less because they had had much less in-patient treatment in the past. As the authors observe, those who have had no prior hospitalization can hardly show a 'further reduction'.

In a study by Gudeman et al (1985) all patients believed to require hospitalisation were admitted instead to a day hospital, in the Massachusetts Mental Health Center. For those without an appropriate living situation there is an inn providing temporary residence from 4pm until 8am. Patients too ill for this service are transferred to in-patient care. Two in-patient services existed before this service was implemented. The study period covered 19 months before and 19 months after the service change. In the period before the change there were 1114 admissions, and 1126 after (23% were involuntary in both periods). Patients were demographically similar.

The porportion of patients receiving day care rose from 19% before the service change to 72% afterwards. The number requiring nighttime residential care was reduced from 81% to 56% and the median length of illness episode (from admission to discharge) decreased 20%. The readmission rate remained the same (18%). There was no increase in suicides, use of medical emergency services or security emergencies.(involving the police). There was a 58% reduction in the use of seclusion, and the rate of seclusion per hour halved.

The cost of providing the service was reduced by 13.5%. There was a corresponding decrease in the number of staff (15.6 %) (because less twenty-four hour care was needed). The savings are almost certainly attributable to this fact. The cost data are not described, and it would appear that only direct costs were used.

Technical efficiency in community services

We have been able to find only one study which looks in detail at the technical efficiency of community services. Frank & Taube (1987) observed that, in 1980, Federally funded CMHCs were responsible for 29% of out-patient visits (2.6 million admissions). Many other non-Federally funded extra-mural care services exist, and these 'free-standing' out-patient services accounted for 43% of out-patient visits in the same year. They examined the differences in performance between centralised and decentralised services, and private and publicly funded clinics. They compared the variations in output (defined in terms of individual patient visits and group visits to the service) with variations in input (defined in terms of physician, nurse and others' (psychologists and social workers) hours; administrative personnel hours; and capital costs (including depreciation)). They used log-transformations of each variable. They included a measure of case-mix, which was the proportions of attendersin groups other than the adult mentally ill as the reference group. These groups were for alcoholics, drug addicts, children, and people with mental handicaps.

The questions they addressed were: are clinics with satelite facilities more productive than centralised clinics?; is private care more efficient than public care? That is, which clinics minimize input mixes, which have lower levels of organisational slack, and which are X-inefficient?

755 of 1,473 clinics presented complete data. They found that the marginal cost curve was upward sloping, i.e. there were decreasing returns to scale. These were of the order of .59. In other words doubling the inputs would result in only a 59% increase in output. With inputs held constant, private facilities produced higher outputs than County facilities, and decentralised clinics produced 12% more visits than centralised clinics. The authors note that when alcoholics were heavily represented in a clinic population, more patient visits resulted.

They make the observation that ignoring case-mix measures does result in an under estimate of the returns to scale, but that this underestimation is small (Feldstein, 1984). They argue that, 'in the presence of ever-decreasing returns to scale one can produce more output by organising the clinic into a number of smaller organizationally linked facilities rather than in a larger single facility organisation'.

On the whole, clinics tended to hire more physicians, relative to other clinical staff 'than would be dictated by cost-minimization'. Out-patient clinics tended to hire more administrative staff relative to physicians than is consistent with cost minimzation. Scheffler and Rossiter (1983) include information which suggests that, there are too many 'other' CMHC workers relative to the number of physicians, and that too few aides are used, relative to physician time. Frank & Taube suggest that their data show too few nurses relative to psychologists and social workers, too many administrative and other treatment staff, and slightly more physicians than is needed to minimize costs. They conclude that, 'there appear to be substantial gains possible from the relocation of personnel'.

They do point out that cost minimization levels do not depend upon output levels, and presumably the reverse is true, that cost minimization does not maximise the efficiency of outputs. This is because productivity is an intervening variable. They did find that there was some evidence (using the Cobb-Douglas model, but not when they used the 'transcendental' model) that state clinics showed some X-inefficiency, and produced 15% fewer visits for the same inputs. However, it is important to bear in mind that they were using 'intermediate' rather than 'final' outputs, in other words they were using the number of clinic visits as an indicator of performance, and assuming that it is an adequate indicator of final outputs, such as the level of patient improvement or satisfaction, or social functioning. This may well not be the case.

The study was also limited to what they called free-standing out-patient clinics of various sorts, and while some of these would qualify as community mental health services, and as CMHCs according to some definitions, the Federally funded CMHCs were excluded from consideration. Nevertheless, given these limitations, the study does produce some thought-provoking findings, many of which could apply elsewhere. Further studies of this sort, using better output measures, are called for.

Cost-benefit studies in community services

Because of the paucity of research in this area we have included the following studies which have a direct bearing on the costs of providing care in the community, or in non-hospital settings. Some of the studies, although not conducted in CMHCs took place in very similar circumstances. Wiesbrod et al (1980) for instance, (see below), describe a community service in which peripatetic staff meet twice a day in a rented house which is the community service headquarters. This might well be described in the UK as a mental health centre, and would certainly be called a mental health service (Huxley et al, 1987).

Murphy and Datel (1976) projected the costs and benefits for 52 discharged patients over a ten year period. The patients were discharged from hospital in Virginia and were subject to the Service Integration for Deinstitutionalisation (SID) model. This consisted of professional assessment and prescription teams, broker-advocates, an automated information system, a quality control team, and a committee of commissioners.

This study has several major deficiencies, not least of which is that the 52 patients were not randomly selected for study, and those who failed to be maintained in the community were dropped from the analysis. It is instructive from other points of view.

The costs measured were the costs of community support services, housing and subsistence, staff costs, deinstitutionalisation costs, and lost economic productivity. Costs to the community in terms of the social and personal consequences of placement of mentally ill people in the neighborhood were not assigned a monetary value. Indirect costs included an overhead rate (65%), an inflation rate, a discount rate (8%), and a rate to cover administrative rather than direct care tasks (40%).

The benefits measured were the savings of institutional costs, ansd increased economic activity. The improvements in patient well-being and increased public awareness of mental illness were not assigned monetary values. The projected costs over ten years were based on the client's previous cost history during time in the community; the broker-advocate's prediction of future needs; and where these were not sufficient, comparison with similar clients.

Before considering the results of this analysis it is worth indicating the limited nature of the direct costs considered and the failure to specify the type of institutional cost (average or marginal) used. In addition, the 52 patients were by no means homogeneous. They were divided into three housing, three employability and three income maintenance groups. One third were in intensive care facilities, one third in intermediate care and one third living independently. Half were employable in sheltered settings and nearly 60% were on state benefit. The figures which relate to individual categories of patient are not given, and some of the cells must have had very small numbers in them.

In only one of the categories of patient did the costs outweigh the benefits. The group involved were ten patients who were in intensive care facilities, were unemployable and received half their income from public sources. The average net cost of maintaining each of these patients in the community for ten years was $400.

In the other categories the benefit-to-cost ratios ranged from 1.52 to 11.86. The authors report that the overall benefit-cost ratio was 1.98, and the average net benefit per client was $20,800 over the ten year period. This net benefit seems to have been achieved by a comparison with the average in-patient cost. There are at least two major probems with this method of calculation. First, we have seen that the 52 patients do not include those who failed to survive in the community and so the costs for the surviving group are underestimated. Second, if the cost measurement for in-patients had been the marginal rather than the average cost then the comparison with the community group would not have been so favourable.

Given the serious shortcomings of this study one can not conclude as the authors do that, 'placing and maintaining clients in the community is desirable from a cost-benefit point of view'.

Wiesbrod et al (1980) conducted an economic benefit-cost analysis of Training in Community Living (TCL), an experimental program, involving peripatetic community mental health workers. It is noteworthy because it is one of the few studies reported by an economist. Further discussion by economists can be found in Marks et al (1988).

The costs assessed were: direct treatment costs; indirect costs - to social service agencies, other hospitals, sheltered workshops, other community agencies, and private medical providers; law enforcement costs; maintenance costs - governemental cash payments, patient payments, experimental centre payments; in kind food and lodgings costs; private and voluntary agency costs;

family burden costs - lost earnings, physical and emotional strain ; illegal activity costs -number of arrests and number of arrests for felony; mortality costs from suicide and natural causes.

Benefits included earnings; labour market behaviour - days of competitive employment, sheltered employment, % days missed from the job, the number of detrimental job changes; improved consumer decision making - represented by patients' insurance expenditure, and the % having a savings account.

These were compared with the costs and benefits of the hospital treatment, in terms of operating costs, capital costs, and a 9% rate of return on plant and land. Experimental costs used were those which reflected the mid-point of the programme to avoid start-up costs, staff learning on the job and early overstaffing. The overall conclusions of the comparison were: that the total costs of treating patients are high, $7200 per patient per year; that between 40 and 50% of costs are indirect costs; that the experimental programme involves higher direct treatment costs, but all other costs are lower; that the experimental programme doubles work productivity; and that the added benefits (which come largely (86%) from the economic productivity of patients in work) amount to 400 dollars more than added costs.

This study raises a number of interesting and important questions. It is worth noting that the comparison between the services may not be entirely fair since the costs of the plant and land are included for the mental hospital, but the 'start up costs' for TCL are ommitted. If included this would mean the TCL costs would be even greater. Although the authors report that the clinical symptoms are less in the TCL patients and their satisfaction both higher, and improving more over time, no data are reported in this paper.

Weisbrod et al, unlike some other authors include 'maintenance costs' even though these are often regarded as 'transfer payments'. They include them because they 'were used subsequently ' for food, clothing and shelter. They also point out that more independent living results in more maintenance costs, and that maintenance costs in hospital save on maintenance costs which the patient would incur if in the community. Different results are obtained if one decides to count costs or benefits that what would otherwise be treated as transfer payments.

Dickey et al (1986) used a refined version of Weisbrod's model in a study of 43 patients with long-standing disability. The average cost per patient for two years service was $67,550. The direct care and treatment costs accounted for 95% of the costs. Individual costs varied considerably, from $24,00 to $99,000. Only 30% of this variation in cost was explained by patient characteristics, and Dickey et al, like many others, are forced to conclude that 'patient condition is not sufficient to explain the variation in the cost of treatment.'

Weisbrod et al wisely make the point that, "unless costs are defined and measured comprehensively, one treatment mode may appear to be less costly than another when in reality that mode merely shifts costs into forms that have not been measured." Williams & Anderson (1975) make the same point with regard to what is called **'social efficiency'**. They point out that the measurement of costs should extend to 'all resources or inputs, and not just one 'key' one, nor even just those which have to be paid for out of the agency's own budget. The main conceptual blockage in the way of sensible and relevant efficiency analysis in the social services is the failure to realise this simple truth.'

Cost-effectiveness studies in community services

May (1970;1971) examined the costs of providing hospital care for psychiatric patients. He points out that cost per diem and cost per case can be misleading. Even pooled estimates of average cost per case based on average length of stay are still not satisfactory since a hospital admits a wide variety of patients, and unless the different case mix is taken into account then one may not be comparing like with like. Wadsworth et al (1957) found that total costs per case were in the same rank order in three hospitals, as per diem costs. When the patients' loss of earnings was included the hospital with the highest per diem cost had the lowest cost per case, because patients were transferred to the community more quickly. Jones et al (1961) produced a similar result without taking the loss of earnings factor into account.

McMahon (1985) reports a method of removing the case-mix problem in studies which compare length of stay. Each patient's length of stay is converted into a percentile score of the population of patients with the same medical condition and age.

Kane et al (1974;1976) examined the cost-effectiveness of different modes of care for patients in 13 medium-level nursing home in Salt Lake City. The patients were randomly allocated to three groups receiving care from: medical and nurse practitioner; medical and nurse practitioner and social worker; and a modified control group with existing medical personnel to which was added the services of a social worker. Costs of project and nonproject input were recorded. The combined care was more effective and cheaper, the savings coming from reduced hospitalisation and related medical costs. The costs were given as annual averages. Hidden costs were neglected, as were costs to other constituencies.

Fenton et al (1984) conducted a two year follow-up of 155 patients randomly assigned to a home or hospital treatment condition. Hospital care was more expensive over the two year period. Fenton et al found, as Kane (above) and Hafner (below) did, that a substantial part of the manpower and operating costs of the home based service was accounted for by periods of hospitalisation.

Dick et al (1985) examined whether day hospital care offered a clinically effective alternative to inpatient care for neurosis, personality disorder and adjustment reactions. They compared a mixed ward (21 bed), two female wards (20 beds each) and a male ward (11 beds) with Roseangle day hospital (a 25 place acute treatment unit). There were two trained staff per shift in each setting, 2-4 consultant sessions per week in each setting an occupational therapist in the day hospital and less than half an occupational therapist in the inpatient setting. The study sample was collected over a 30 month period and new patients were randomised to early transfer to the day setting.

The authors argue that only relative costs were of interest, i.e. not those which pertain to both services. Transfer payments were excluded, ' as these do not constitute resource costs but transfers from one sector of society to another'. They used average ward costs as a proxy for marginal costs after a brief exercise to see whether study patients consumed the same amount of staff time. The authors point out that this exercise involved only a small number of patients and was not sufficiently large to justify applying to all the study patients, but for the purpose of this paper they then do so!

There were 334 relevant admissions between January 1980 and December 1981. 62 were discharged before being seen, and a number of others were missed. 242 remained to be interviewed or discussed. 39 were 'too well' (sic) and 101 too ill to be included. 27 refused, leaving 75 suitable and willing. 16 more patients were recruited in 1982. 48 patients were randomly allocated to continued inpatient care and 43 to day care. At 4 months 45 of the former and 38 of the latter we re-interviewed.

The overall levels of severity of disorder in the two groups did not differ, but the decrease in severity for day patients was significantly greater at 4 but not at 12 months. There were no significant differences in the use of medication. More of the hospital subjects were admitted and used emergency services but the differences were not significant.

Costs were lower for the day patients because of, a single shift day, the lower number of nurses in training and half the number of junior doctor hours. The cost per patient day was: DGH wards - 11.78; mental hospital wards - 9.07; and Roseangle 2.94. The average cost per case for nursing and junior doctor services was 365.10, 272.10, and 111.72 respectively.

The author notes (but then ignores the fact) that because one cannot make staffing reductions on wards, which are pro rata with reductions in the number of inpatient days, marginal and average cost are not the same thing. A further potential weakness of the study is that the 'home costs' were derived from the Family Expenditure survey of 1981, and may not have been an accurate reflection of the costs to these patients. Because the same method was used in relation to each patient group this does not effect the comparison of relative costs. Given the clinical equivalence of patients the day service was more cost effective at 65% of the hospital costs.

Hafner (1985) reports on the implementation of a new community mental health care system in Mannheim. In the early years of the introduction of this service there was a sharp increase in total service utilization, from 9.5/1000 of the population in 1974 to 19.3/1000 in 1980. We will return to this finding, (which is repeated in other countries) in the section on target efficiencies below. Hafner adds that the high utilization rate, combined with the fact that providers had frequently to refuse care for minor cases indicates that this effect was 'not reached by meeting all needs but by the saturation of service capacity'. He also notes that there was also a true change in the amount of morbidity during this period, due to increases in alcohol related illness and parasuicides.

The community service (called the 'complementary care system') comprised group homes and sheltered housing, outpatient care, patient clubs and 'lay initiatives'. The rate of treated cases of schizophrenia increased 'parallel to the augmentation of places offered by sheltered homes and group homes'. The sharp rise in the number of treated episodes is attributed to the growing number of discharges of long-stay patients. 60% of long stay patients and 75% of patients admitted with episodes of disorder go into complementary care rather than into hospital. The most frequent care combinations outside hospital are sheltered workshop plus out-patient care, and home plus out-patient care. These most frequent combinations are not, however, very frequent , accounting for only 11% and 10% respectively. This demonstrates the range of possible combinations of care. Hafner argues that, 'in comparable cases an extensive utilization of complementary care reduces the possibility of admission to hospital.'

In reporting on the costs of this service Hafner only reports direct costs of contacts with facilities. Only 7 out of 145 discharged patients incurred higher costs than would have resulted from long term treatment in the mental hospital. Almost 80% of the costs accrue from hospital stays in the community group (see Kane et al above).

Modified cost-benefit and cost-effectiveness analysis

Goldberg (Glass & Goldberg 1977;Goldberg & Jones, 1980; Goldberg, 1983; Hyde et al ,1987) has attempted to provide answers to some of the problems encountered in other cost-benefit and cost-effectiveness studies in this field. He has de-

91

veloped a modified form of cost-benefit analysis in which the service effects which cannot be expressed in financial terms are called 'soft' costs. If a service which produces more soft costs is also cheaper it is said to **dominate** the other service. Weisbrod et al implicitly used this model.

In his 1980 study Goldberg includes soft costs, but also extends the costing exercise to local authority and voluntary services provided in the community, avoiding the problem identified by Williams. This study was a 10-12 year follow-up of first admission schizophrenia sufferers, and compared the performance of the mental hospital with a District General Hospital (DGH) unit. Weaknesses in the costing exercises in this study were that hospital records were used to estimate costs; the inpatient costs were for all patients not just the schizophrenia sufferers; and capital costs were excluded.

Goldberg uses unit costs, which, he argues, are equivalent to long run marginal costs excluding capital costs, and are also opportunity costs in the sense that these resources could have been used elsewhere. He excludes transfer payments.

The DGH was superior in terms of costs for three main reasons. The length of stay was shorter; the local authority costs were higher for mental hospital patients because their children went into care in group homes rather than cheaper foster care; and the DGH unit patients earned more, and fewer family members have to give up work to look after them.

Soft costs also favour the DGH. These include: the number of in-patient days; fewer changes in drugs; less impaired sociability; greater employability; and fewer strange postures. Soft benefits also favour the DGH, in terms of: greater sociability; heterosexual performance; weeks employed; drive, constructiveness and realism at work; leisure; and marital adjustment.

Another study (Jones and Goldberg, 1980) compared a cohort which had been ill for 3-4 years. Unit costs were greater in the DGH because of the large number of professional staff (this is a teaching unit), but the overall economic effect favoured the DGH. Goldberg asserts that, 'this part of the study therefore confirmed Fein's view that one might cost society less by spending more'.

Hyde et al (1987) report on the use of the modified cost-benefit analysis on two groups of patients, one in a hostel ward and the other in hospital. The groups of patients were matched and assigned to the hostel-ward on the toss of a coin. The non-financial effects (the soft costs) were problem behaviours, clinical state, socially adaptive and useful behaviours, time budget and satisfaction with living conditions. Average daily costs per patient and average annual costs regardless of location were calculated. The first covers NHS costs only but the second also includes local authority and Home Office costs. Capital costs were included using a discount rate of 5%, evaluation costs were excluded, service costs were recorded, rates, electricity, maintenance,and food were included. Costs were also included for time spent in local authority accommodation (based on the possibly unreliable CIPFA rates for 1983) and time spent in prison. Transfer payments were excluded.

The capital costs for the hostel ward were less than for the hospital ward, but formed only a small proportion of the costs (10 and 15% respectively). Nursing costs were 60% of the costs of the hostel ward, and 31% of the hospital costs. The hospital patients seemed to continue to acquire psychotic impairments compared with the hostel ward residents. The latter developed superior domestic skills, used more facilities in the community and were more likely to engage in constructive activities. The cost of providing care in the hostel ward was less than in the hospital ward, at 10,284 per patient/year, compared with 11,504. If the eight patients who did not have to be admitted to the hospital are matched with their hospital counterparts the cost for the hostel ward is 9,240 per patient/year.

The authors point out that the research team were also the evaluators and although standardised assessments were used to reduce bias, the service providers were not blind. The study concerns a small number of patients which makes generalisation difficult, but these patients were the total available in the service from a ten year accumulation. Although the nursing costs were high in the hostel ward, these were offset by the reduction in general service costs. The savings made by moving patients to the hostel ward are only likely to apply where the DGH unit is the alternative; where the mental hospital is the alternative costs may already be lower than the hostel ward, and the disabled mental hospital patients would require just as much if not more nursing care if transferred to a community setting such as a hostel ward.

The impact of economic cut-backs

A small number of papers refer to the increasing funding difficulties facing CMHCs. This is partly due to the lack of Federal support, but also to the economic recession. Ochberg (1976) predicted that, as a result of legislative trends, centres would be forced to devote increasing time and effort to financial concerns. Edwards & Mitchell (1987) identified four effective strategies for confronting declining financial resources These were: increased efficiency; increased efforts to obtain fee for service; more economical modes of treatment; and finally, service reduction. Winslow (1982) also advocates more competitive marketing of services, and argues that the staff need to be 'reprofessionalized'. The decline in the use of CMHCs as training centres needs to be reversed. Woy et al (1981) suggest that those centres which maximise their earnings by concentrating on traditional services, are more likely to survive than those who try to maintain all their services. Pardes & Stockdill (1984) recommend the use of business techniques.

Goplerud et al (1983) used a panel of expert informants to produce 77 strategies for surviving cut-backs. McLaughlin & Zelman (1987) discuss the potential of entrepreneurship in CMHCs, the technical assistance required from the management, and the need to devolve some aspects of financial control.

Efficiency and hidden morbidity

Very little consideration has been given to the benefits which accrue from the recognition and treatment of hidden morbidity. The study by Johnstone & Goldberg (1976) will be referred to below (Effectiveness chapter), and is perhaps the only study to demonstrate the benefits to patients in general practice, of having a disorder which would have remained hidden, identified. The costs associated with not correctly identifying and then treating a psychiatric problem are made up of two elements. There is the benefit, which is foregone, of having the correct treatment. The patients in Johnstone & Goldberg whose GHQ scores were not revealed to the GP tended to recover more slowly, and this delay presumably had personal, social and possibly economic costs. The second cost element is that which results from inappropriate and unnecessary consultation, investigation and treatment which could have been avoided had the hidden disorder been recognised. Goldberg points out that we do not know what the effect on a health service would be if screening was introduced, but he thinks that it is important that we find out. Assuming that further studies can show that intervention with cases identified by screening instruments is cost-effective, the benefits to the patient and to the health service are likely to be considerable.

Funding differences in the US and UK

As we have noted elsewhere in this book, there are substantial similarities between the US and the UK in terms of the problems which social policy makers face in providing community services. We have also noted the growing tendency for funding of health care in the UK to become more like funding in the US. Fundamental differences remain however, and recent changes in funding strategies in the US can inform the planning of services in the UK.

Changes in Medicare reimbursement for elderly people, from retrospective cost based reimbursement to a prospective payment system, based on national average costs for 460 diagnostic related groups, is instructive. This has radically altered the incentives for providing service. Under the old scheme there waas reimbursement of all items of service, and therefore an incentive to consume resources. Under the new scheme there is a disincentive to go beyond national average costs, because this extra expenditure will not be reimbursed.

McGuire & Fairbank (1988) compared psychiatric service use in a fee for service system and a Health Maintenance Organisation (HMO). The probability that a non-user would become a user is the same in the fee for service and HMO systems, but the probability of continuing is less in the HMO than in the fee for service system. The authors do not give data relating to the nature of the service visits in the fee for service system, so it is not possible to say whether this additional service was necessary or unnecessary.

Taube & Burns (1988) show that psychiatric DRGs are not good predictors of use of service (Taube et al, 1984), nor are patient characteristics as recorded in patient notes (Jencks et al, 1987). Severity, type of hospital (Horn et al 1986; Freiman et al 1987) and type of clinic (Frank & Taube, 1987) are related to use, but social and area characteristics are better indicators of use (Brandon, 1975; Jencks et al, 1987). These findings exactly parallel findings in the prediction of the outcome of episodes of illness, where social variables are related to outcome, but diagnosis is not (see Goldberg & Huxley, 1980) (see also concluding chapter).

Target efficiencies in CMHCs

We have already considered the original purposes of CMHCs, and noted that these included an attempt, albeit ill-defined, to improve the horizontal target efficiency of mental health services. This was to be achieved by targeting disadvantaged groups of various sorts.

The intention also was to change the balance of care towards the community and away from the institution, in part by providing a wider range of services which were more accessible. This was bound to imply an increase in the numbers of people served, although this does not appear to have been a stated intention of the US government. The objectives were couched more in terms of the transfer of care, rather than its enhanced efficiency.

Conceptual issues

We have seen above that services need to be specific about their target population. Once the targets have been specified, then the extent to which the target population is served is a useful measure of service performance. This is horizontal target efficiency referred to earlier in this chapter. If the service has been set up to provide for patients with long-term rather than short-term problems, or specifically to help schizophrenia sufferers, then the extent to which the users of the service are from these groups is another useful indicator of efficiency. This is vertical target efficiency.

The use of these concepts highlights the importance of several factors which we may otherwise take for granted, or ignore. Firstly, it is clear that the target populations must be specified, and that when this is done clearly, we can have greater confidence when we compare different services; we would obviously find it difficult to directly compare services whose target groups are very different. This 'case-mix' problem has been referred to above.

Secondly, changes in vertical and horizontal target efficiency (over time), are of considerable interest. Examining these changes is one of the ways in which the impact of new services can be monitored. Monitoring of this sort may also raise the question, for service providers, of whether they should alter the criteria for acceptance into the service in order to increase use by the target group, or change the target group altogether.

Thirdly, studies of target efficiency make use of service contact as the unit of analysis. Inpatient or extra-mural episodes of care are more than simply contacts with service, and for some purposes different units of analysis may be preferable. Taube & Burns (1988) have suggested that treatment category units match clinical decision making and resource utilisation better than traditional disgnostic categories.

Fourthly, the concepts help to emphasise that the task of providing a service is a function of both the ability of the service to 'find' the right cases in the population, and the ability to use appropriate techniques for 'screening out' people who are not eligible for service. The major failures of generic social work departments in the UK in the 1970s was the inability to grasp these fundamental distinctions (and to take so long to find ways of making them operational); there are signs that these lessons have been learned (Challis & Davies, 1986).

On a methodological note, we are using the terms 'case-finding' and 'screening' in the way Challis and Davies (1986) use them rather than in the way advocated by Williams (1986). We use 'epidemiological surveys' in the same way as Williams, but when we refer to 'case-finding' we mean **the process whereby a service is used by, or reaches, the target population.** We use 'screening' to mean **the process whereby those reaching the service are judged to be 'eligible' to receive it.** We realise that these usages are not the same as those advocated in medicine (Sackett & Holland, 1975) and hope that we do not add to terminological confusion by adopting them.

The main means of assessing the target efficiency of a service is by monitoring the frequency and type of referral. The study of 'utilization rates' does not, on its own, give a complete picture. We also need to know the expected rate of disorder in the particular population being served, and we need to know the service targets. We may also need to know the social and demographic characteristics of the population, especially if the target groups represent minorities within the population, such as ethnic minorities, or lower-income groups. Nowadays much better census data is available, much of it at ward level, to enable us to relate services to population characteristics. On the whole there are more proponents of this approach, (which is, broadly speaking, 'social indicator' analysis) (e.g. Mustian & See, 1973; DeWitt-Kay, 1978; Warheit et al, 1978; Struening, 1983) than opponents (Cochran 1979). It is worth noting that efficiency judgements are technical ones, they do not tell us which groups to target, or how we should alter our services in order to improve efficiency.

The target efficiencies can be related to both incidence and prevalence of disorder in the community. To assess horizontal target efficiency the incidence of new cases in the community would be compared with the rate of new cases seen in the service. The prevalence of cases in the community would be compared with the total number seen by the service over the same period. (It would be essential for the definitions of a 'new' episode, and of a 'chronic' case to be comparable in both the survey and the service).

Vertical target efficiency would be assessed in relation to the specific target group for the service. In the case of a psychiatric service, which presumably aims to serve 'cases', one would look at the proportion of the total cases seen over a specific time which were 'cases' according to diagnostic criteria. If the service is aimed at acute disorder then one would want to see what proportion of the total number of cases were suffering from acute episodes. (In epidemiological terms these are issues of sensitivity and specificity). High target efficiencies depend upon the adequacy of **both** case-finding **and** screening, or assessment, techniques.

There are, of course many other influences upon the efficiency of a service. Of particular importance are the nature of the total mixture of services available, and the health care policies of the responsible administrative authorities (see, for example, Goodban et al, 1987). For instance, Goldberg and Huxley (1980), referring to data from psychiatric case registers (which, they point out, is the best source of data about the distribution of mental illness as described by psychiatrists) show that the outpatient contacts in Salford and Camberwell differed from one another by six standard deviations (from the national average). The more liberally staffed Camberwell service looked after a substantially larger number of people suffering from depression, but an equal number of people suffering from schizophrenia.

They conclude, "it seems likely that over the nation the existing out-patient services are not prevented from seeing their schizophrenic patients by shortage of resources. However, it seems likely that additional resources would allow psychiatric services to meet the needs of patients with depression and with psychological problems related to physical disease".

In a period of expanding resources between 1965 and 1970 the reported prevalence of schizophrenia remained constant, but there was an increase in those treated for personality disorder, alcoholism and marital problems (Wing & Hailey, 1972). These issues will be reconsidered, briefly, later in this review.

Horizontal target efficiency

Estimates of the levels of morbidity in the population are essential in order to examine horizontal target efficiency. Information is needed from reliable community surveys. Fortunately these are becoming increasingly available, and the results tend to confirm Goldberg and Huxley's (1980) assertion that there is now more agreement than disagreement about the incidence and prevalence of disorder in the community. The social factors which give rise to variations in incidence and prevalence are also receiving more attention (see for example, Brandon (1975)). It is not possible to describe all this work in detail here, and it would be wrong to pretend that questions of the definition and measurement of disorder are finally resolved.

A brief review of recent work suggests, however, that:

(i) Depression in the community is a prevalent disorder, and much of it is of the same severity as treated depression in outpatient settings, and that much of the depression in the community is not treated (Katon,1987; Brown & Craig, 1986; Weissman, 1987)

(ii) Treated prevalence (6 month) is about 6-7% of the population (Shapiro et al,1984; Bebbington et al, 1981; Hodiamont et al 1987)

(iii) Higher risk groups include women, lower class men, unemployed, divorced widowed and separàted (Hodiamont et al 1987; Yates, 1986; Finlay-Jones & Burvill, 1977)

(iv) Annual period prevalence is about 25% (Goldberg & Huxley, 1980; Reynolds, 1981)

(v) Anxiety disorders have a prevalence of about 3%, panic disorders also about 3% and about 6% of the consulting population (Katon, 1987; Reich, 1986)

(vi) The services are underutilized by various groups in the community, such as ethnic minorities and the poor (Brandon 1975).

This knowledge should enable us to be increasingly specific about the expected rates of disorder in a population, within broad limits, and taking into account the socio-demographic and social area characteristics which would affect the rates of disorder and help-seeking behaviour.

We can make an estimation of the horizontal target efficiency of a service against these expected figures. This would be of most value over time, so that the effects of changes in the administration of the service could be monitored. One must bear in mind that the aim of the service is not to serve all those in need, but rather, within the limits of scarce resources, to serve as many as possible , in defined groups, as efficiently as possible.

It is difficult to assess the impact of the CMHCs on the **total** psychiatric service, and it may be easier to take certain aspects, such as institutional admissions, and look at the impact on these, more manageable, statistics. The impact on state hospital admission is difficult to disentangle from the effects of the policy of deinstitutionalisation which was a contemporary development (Schaeffer et al ,1978; Allessi & Wecht, 1976). Windle and Scully (1976) reported that, in a study of 16 states over 5 years, those with CMHCs had state admission rates which declined or increased less, than those without, but that state hospital **resident** rates were unchanged.

Windle et al (1987) attempted to assess the impact of federally funded CMHCs on the quantity and range of mental health services, by matching 63 catchment areas in which CMHCs began to receive federal funding in 1974-5 with areas which never received federal CMHC funding. The average increases in amounts of service, numbers of staff, expenditures, and availability and accessibility of services were compared. They argue that the establishment of local CMHCs did have an impact on the quantity, availability and the accessibility of services. No cost data are reported, and no data regarding the effectiveness of services.

One confounding problem in investigations of this sort, is the level of true morbidity in the population. If this changes substantially, then an increase in the number of cases seen could be due to this real increase, rather than to an improvement in the case-finding ability of the new service. This is a phenomenon observed by Hafner (1985) in West Germany, where there has been (as there has elsewhere) a real increase in morbidity related to alcohol and parasuicide.

A paper by Lehman will help to illustrate some of these points. Lehman et al (1984) examined the rates of annual treated prevalence and annual treated incidence between the mid sixties and the early 1970s. They defined chronic disorders as those which required three hospitalisations in a year, or 365 consecutive days of treatment during the five study years. The admission data which they used was obtained from the Monroe County

Case Register between 1964 and 1970.

During this period the annual treated incidence of chronic disorders remained very much the same at .47 per 1000 in 1964 and .41 per 1000 in 1970. The annual treated incidence of non-chronic disorders rose during the same period by 37% (p<.001). Similarly, the annual treated prevalence of chronic cases remained the same (at .6%) but the annual treated incidence rose by 43%, from 1.4 to 1.9% in 1970 (p<.01). Lehman makes the point that this period coincides with the development of the CMHCs. We can be fairly certain that, even if there was an increase in true morbidity during this period, that it was not of the order of 40%, and that service developments which occurred at the time did play a large part in this increase. The rates of increase varied by diagnostic group and by area of origin.

We cannot say whether these results represent an improvement in target efficiency since we do not know whether the service aimed to meet the needs of people with less chronic disorders. If it did, then this may represent an improvement. The results do not allow us to say anything about the technical efficiency of the delivery of the service, which may have been provided at an increased unit cost per patient. In addition we could not be sure, without looking at the total service, whether these increases represented a transfer of care from another, and presumably declining, service area.

In order to assess horizontal target efficiency we need to know, from community surveys how many people with episodes of disorder actually reach the services. Shapiro et al (1984) report on the use of mental health services by non-institutionalised adults, in the NIMH Epidemiological Catchment Area Program (ECA). Disorder was assessed using the Diagnostic Interview Schedule (DIS). The appropriateness of the DIS has been questioned because of a less than adequate relationship with clinical judgement (Robins et al,1982; Helzer et al, 1985), but its use has been defended in community surveys (Erdman et al, 1987). In each of the study areas a wide range of services was provided, including CMHCs.

The results show that people who have a recent DIS disorder are more likely to make a mental health visit than those with a past DIS disorder. The proportion of patients with a visit for a physical or emotional problem was high, the median in all three sites was 67%. The rates for antisocial personality disorder, affective disorder and schizophrenia were similar (about 80%). One third of those who consulted had no DIS disorder. This does not necessarily mean that they were not 'ill', because of the imperfect relationship between the DIS and clinical judgement. Although large numbers of patients were 'found' by the service, there were still a large proportion who were not; nearly 40% of the substance abusers did not consult during the previous 6 months. The proportion of patients who saw a mental health specialist ranged from 24 to 38%. The number of mental health specialists was greatest in New Haven, and this was where the consultation rate with specialists was highest.

Leaf et al (1985) report somewhat similar results from Yale, where over half of the schizophrenia sufferers and those with 'somatisation' had mental health contacts, but the rates for alcoholism was only 12.7%, and 13.2% for drug abusers. They report that the factors most strongly associated with help seeking, in the prior 6 months, are not the same as those which are correlated with frequency of contact among service users. The individual's perception of their mental health and the existence of a DIS disorder are the two factors most strongly associated with help seeking.

Brandon (1975) examined the impact of CMHCs on service use in New York, and the effect on utilisation rates. He examined the extent to which social area characteristics (SAC) (income, race,age,sex,housing and family structure) and facility coverage (FC) (emergency rooms, twenty-four hour hospitalisation,partial hospitalisation, out-patient facilities, and consultation and education services) contributed to the variation in utilisation rates. He was able to compare areas with and without CMHCs. He used consultation rates based on both health areas (24,000) and catchment areas (approximately 200,000). He found that there was a systematic relationship between SAC and utilisation rates, which explained 54% of the variance in the out-patient rate, and 44% of the variance of the inpatient rates. In order to assess whether these results simply reflected different facility coverage, he entered FC into the regression analysis. Only 7% more of the variance of utilisation was explained. Reversing the procedure, and entering FC into the analysis first resulted in less explanatory power than when SAC was entered first (32% of the variance of out-patient rates and 18% of the variance of inpatient rates). He concludes that ' only 7% of out-patient rate variance and 6% of inpatient are explained by facility coverage, independently of social area characteristics'.

In all health districts there was a positive and significant relationship between inpatient and out-patient utilisation rates. The ratio was consistent. Taking this to be an indication of the balance of service provision between institutional and extra-mural care Brandon examined the impact on this ratio of the presence of CMHCs, which were introduced with the intention of altering this balance. He found that coverage by a CMHC has no effect on the positive correlation between in and out-patient utilisation rates. In New York, he concludes, 'persons with no prior service enter both in and out-patient services at a high or low rate that is only partly dependent on social variables and hardly dependent on facility location...about 5% of the variance in either inpatient or out-patient rates is due to a residual propensity to use service'.

The effect of CMHC coverage seems to be to strongly increase the clinic utilisation rate, moderately increase the hospitalisation rate but not affect the ratio between the two. Providing a comprehensive service at a hospital or clinic site will not necessarily reduce the rate of hospitalisation. Before considering some of the other interesting results of this study, we should point out that these particular findings bear a striking resemblance to those reported by Boardman et al (1987) in the UK. This similarity will be described later. Similar results have been reported in Canada and in New Zealand. Miller et al (1986) constructed a model for predicting use of psychiatric services. They applied this model which included age, educational level, employment status, type of residence to the rates of disorder in 1976 and 1980, and found that 'the model demonstrates a relation between utilization rates and sociodemographic indicators, and that these indicators are stable over time.' Hall (1988) in New Zealand studied the use of four community based centres and found that various combinations of demographic variables contribute significantly to centre use.

Brandon examines the results for low income groups, and notes that FC explains more variance for low than for high income areas. He says that it may be that lower income persons are drawn to a service which is placed near them, or will travel less distance than higher income persons and so are susceptible to the FC effect. The presence of a large municipal hospital in a health district has the effect of decreasing the out-patient utilisation rates. When municipal out-patient clinics are available to poor people, inpatient hospitalisation rates go down, and where large hospitals are in 'poor' areas the inpatient rate goes up and the out-patient rate goes down. In this study therefore, Brandon suggests that the results indicate that, 'poor people thus receive neither a continuum of service nor an offering of what is appropriate; rather, they get what is placed near them'.

Commenting on the fact that CMHCs are to be found in areas with more young people , fewer blacks, more Puerto Ricans, Italians and Irish, more substandard housing, and where fewer people drive to work, Brandon argues that the actual operation of the mental health service system is affected more by implicit than explicit political decisions. He says,

> an explicit decision would entail promulgation and implementation of a certain type of service program dedicated to announced goals and related to the particular characteristics, needs or desires of the population to be serviced. An implicit relationship may be inferred when, with no such promulgation, we find a consistent relationship between the social characteristics of areas and the type of facilities located in or near those areas. Our finding of prediction of different utilisation rates by the joint action of SAC and FC indicates that such implicit decisions are indeed the major force in mental

health services. Thus when we observe that the CMHC coverage independently explains only 3% of the variance in out-patient admissions, 1% for inpatient, and 0% for the inpatient /out-patient ratio, we must look elsewhere for an explanation. The major factor in utilisation is the distribution of social groups and non-CMHC services. ...when there is a large ongoing system of service (state, municipal, and voluntary hospital) a program strategy based upon awarding grants for creation of alternative projects will not produce any significant change in the pre-existing system.

The impact of these conclusions from one remote service in the USA , might be of little significance, were it not for the following factors: the similarities between the untreated and treated rates of disorder in the USA and the UK are considerable; the social policies of the two governments with respect to health and mental health care are becoming more similar; there are a growing number of community mental health service developments in the UK which are similar in intention to the USA CMHCs; and the focus on care for mentally ill people is shifting towards primary health and social care agencies in both countries. All the more understandable then, that we should find the results of Boardman et al (1987) in the UK, to resemble those reported by Brandon (1975) in the USA, Miller et al (1986) in Canada, and Hall (1988) in New Zealand.

Boardman et al report on the establishment of a multiprofessional team service (MPT), using a walk-in (in addition to the usual) referral system and a crisis intervention team (CIT) added to deal with emergencies which could not get to the centre. The services were provided by the mental health advice centre in Lewisham (Bouras et al, 1982; Boardman et al, 1986). From the inception of the service in 1978, the referrals increased to the MPT, but referrals to the CIT have gone down. The authors suggest that this latter finding may be due to the service staff's increasing experience and change of practice, in particular in filtering out unsuitable cases (or increasing vertical target efficiency; see below.)

For the purpose of this part of the chapter the relevant findings are that the service had no impact on the number of admissions elsewhere in the service. There was a coincidental, but slight decline in the number of out-patient referrals, and a dramatic fall in the number of domiciliary visits. A substantial number of out-patients were referred by the MPT, and when these were removed the slight decline in numbers was observed.

The introduction of the MPT caused an increase in new patient numbers and this increase shows no sign of reaching any plateau.
The authors note a similar tendency elsewhere (Munk-Jorgensen, 1985; Woof et al , 1983; Hafner & Klug, 1982), and that as

103

elsewhere, these patients tend to be suffering from neurotic disorders. They argue that these patients are usually treated in primary care agencies, and that the creation of this specialist service results in a transfer of care from this sector. They cannot demonstrate this hypothesis directly since they do not have figures which relate to the rates of treated disorder by primary care agencies.

Of considerable interest is the fact that inpatient admissions were unaffected by this increase. If Brandon is right, and if one assumes that the inpatient to out-patient ratio is an indicator of the change of the balance of care in a service (which is obviously an over-simplification of the dynamics of the services) then if the service fundamentally alters the balance of provision, then this should be reflected in the inpatient to out-patient ratio. We have analysed the in to out-patient ratios based on the figures given by Boardman et al, and the findings are given below.

Table 4.1 Ratios of in-patient to out-patient referral rates

Year	Out-Patient Ratio	Total Extra-Mural Care Ratio
1978	1:3	1:5
1979	1:2	1:8
1980	1:2	1:16
1981	1:2	1:10
1982	1:1.3	1:8
1983	1:1.3	1:7
1984	1:2	1:11
1985	1:2	1:10
1986	1:2	1:10

(Based on figures given by Boardman et al 1987)

We can see that, over the period since 1978 the ratio of the number of in-patients referred compared to the number of out-patients referred hardly changed, and that the total extra-mural ratio (of out-patients, domiciliary visits etc) increased and then decreased and settled at a reasonably steady rate. However a more reasonable comparison would include data for the ten years prior to the introduction of the service. There is an indication that the ratio of total extra-mural care may have been lower in this period, since it was only 1:5 in 1978. Without this information we are unable to say whether the new service fundamentally altered the pre-existing balance of care. In the next section we look a the way in which this service increased its vertical target efficiency.

Some studies report findings which have a bearing on the utilisation rates of specific target groups in the community. Brandon (1975) refers to the utilisation rates of the poor. Wells et al (1987) report on the underutilization of mental health services by Mexican Americans. This study was part of the ECA research referred to above, and found that underutilization was not explained by a lower prevalence of disorder, or by reliance on forms of 'alternative' medical care. Williams (1986) argues that most post-war studies of the use of services by Afro-Americans under-sample middle class Afro-Americans, and poor, young urban Afro-American males. Even the ECA research is said to be guilty of this error.

Vertical target efficiency

The NIMH (1977) and Herbert (1978) draw attention to the tendency for CMHCs to treat declining proportions of schizo-phrenia sufferers. These authors were, in effect, accusing the CMHCs of having a low target efficiency with regard to schizo-phrenia sufferers. A consistent theme in some parts of the literature, and certainly among many psychiatrists, is the alleged tendency for CMHCs to treat minor morbidity , and to fail to take up a share of the care of people with serious mental illnesses. Worse, the CMHCs came to be equated in some people's minds with the care of the 'worried well'. Langsley (1980) pointed out that in 1975, 20% of CMHC patients were 'not mentally ill' but 'merely socially maladjusted.' On the basis of the literature which relates to vertical target efficiency, we believe that the picture is more complex than this.

It is true that, for instance, between 1970 and 1975 the proportion of all patients who were schizophrenia sufferers went down from 15 to 10 %. However, as Goldman et al (1980) point out, the dilution in the proportion of cases of schizophrenia was due to the increase in new populations of previously untreated patients. Between 1983 and 1986 the total number of patients trebled. The number of schizophrenia sufferers admitted to private hospitals increased 50% during the same time period, while the number seen in out-patient clinics remained the same. The transfer of care is one factor held to be responsible for the findings of Goldman et al (1980). Goldman et al (1980) examined the rates of treatment of schizophrenia sufferers according the the CMHC Inventory. These data are also treated/admission data. As you can see from the figures in Table 4.2 below, the numbers of schizophrenia sufferers in treatment in the CMHCs rose between 1970 and 1975. The state and DGH populations declined, and the private hospital numbers increased.

The number of admissions with a diagnosis of schizophrenia to CMHCs increased 82% between 1970 and 1975 compared with a 1% decrease in admissions to all other facilities. The increase resulted largely from the transfer of patients from other facilities. The figures show that he expansion of out-patient services has not resulted in increased service delivery to schizophrenia sufferers.

The transfer of patients to CMHCs which have been established more recently, is not so marked. This may be because they are not located in mental hospitals , and tend to be smaller than the CMHCs which were established in the early days. Some of the explanation for increases at CMHCs and decline in total number of schizophrenia sufferers in general hospital psychiatric units may have been due to the change in the name of the DGH units to 'Community Mental Health Centre'! This phenomenon might be observed in the UK.

Table 4.2 Changes in numbers of patient by facility

Type of facility	Number with schizophrenia	
	1970	1975
CMHC	50597	91914
OP	148031	148303
Inpatient State & County		
Mental Hospital	146121	143398
Private	18903	28315
DGH	136730	124458
Total	301745	296171
All facilities	500382	536388

(Source: Goldman et al (1980))

If the services were all set up to deal only with schizophrenia. and if admissions were the only service offered, then VTE would be judged by looking at the % of cases who suffer from schizophrenia. If these assumptions were accepted then the CMHCs clearly do worse than the state mental hospitals, for example, as the percentages in the following table (4.3) confirm.

Table 4.3 Schizophrenia sufferers by facility

Type of facility	% of patients with schizophrenia	
	1970	1975
CMHC	15.1	10.0
OP	16.8	10.5
Inpatient		
State & County MH	31.8	33.1
Private	20.7	21.8
DGH	26.3	24.1
Total	28.2	27.5
All facilities	21.9	15.8

(Source: Goldman et al (1980))

Goldman et al caution that admission data on their own are not a complete measure of quantity of service, and do not indicate anything about the intensity or quality of treatment.

According to data from the Salford Case Register, the development of extra-mural injection clinics, and community psychiatric nursing services, appears to increase service use (point-prevalence), but have minimal affect on the use of other services (Woof et al, 1983). Peet (1986) reports an increase in the rates of referrals to consultant psychiatrists following the establishment of a community team in Derbyshire, but notes that the increase only brought a low referral rate up to one more in line with national norms. Hutton (1985) reports an increase in the number of self-referrals during the first three years existence of a community mental health centre. She suggests that these referrals were 'generally appropriate' and were often for 'long-standing emotional distress'.

In a study of the length of stay in a state hospital and a CMHC, Goodban et al (1987) provide details of the different nature of the patient populations involved. The study included all referrals made to the two services during the last 6 months of 1983. When geriatric patients, drug and alcohol abusers, and court mandated admissions were excluded there were 133 left in the hospital sample, and 187 in the CMHC sample. While this represented 67% of the CMHC referrals, it represented only 8% of the state hospital referrals!

Among the differences between the two samples were the following: mean length of stay (shorter in CMHC); (note that median length of stay was similar); range of number of days inpatient status (greater at CMHC); % staying more than 100 days (fewer in CMHC); male:female ratio (higher in hospital); schizophrenia diagnosis (fewer in CMHC); 'other' disorders (higher in CMHC); discharged within the previous 6 months from a psychiatric hospital (lower in CMHC); and in receipt of disability payments for two years or more (lower in CMHC).

The authors attempted to predict the length of stay, using a log-transformation of length of stay. No factors were predictive of length of stay in both settings. In the CMHC diagnosis (of psychosis) was the best predictor (but accounted for only 10% of the variance). In the hospital the disability payment, age (older) and discharge from a psychiatric hospital in the previous six months were all predictors of length of stay (but accounted for only 9% of the variance).

Both services had comparable treatment programmes and admission criteria. Both took 'public' sector patients, and both had access to the same aftercare and community resources. The role of each within the total service was evidently different. This role was shaped by many factors, and many of these were not financial considerations. The need for asylum, past history of reliance upon institutional care, the need for security and structure and for different levels of stimulation, are some of the factors mentioned by Goodban et al. They conclude that 'the hospital's program, as influenced by the role of the facility within a larger system of care, may be a prime and legitimate influence' upon the type of patient referred to and cared for by the hospital.

The findings of this paper confirm the difficulty of comparing parts of the service which fulfil very different needs. We have seen above, that the costs of care vary with the levels of disability of the population served. Solutions providing greater cost-efficiency relative to one type of care may actually be less cost-effective when tested against other types - this is Goldberg's conclusion with regard to hostel wards.

Similarly, one can compare the relative vertical target efficiencies of services which are aiming to deal with different groups of patients, but it would be more useful to compare two services if they were aiming to deal with the same patients, because one could then examine the causes of different efficiency levels, and thus learn something which might help improve service delivery, and efficiency..

Boardman et al (1987) report on the establishment of a multi-professional team (MPT) and a crisis intervention team (CIT). The MPT and the CIT were set up for different purposes. They received referrals from different sources (70% of MPT referrals were from GPs; 47% of CIT). The MPT patients were more likely to be younger, and more frequently suffering from an adjustment reaction (34%). The patients were more often women, in employment, from a Caribbean background, divorced,widowed or separated, and often not known to the psychiatric services. The CIT patients were older, previously known, psychotic, and in need of a domiciliary or admission service. The authors conclude that the services were 'fulfilling the need for which they were set up'. If assessed in relation to specific target groups of patients we would say that the vertical target efficiencies of both services was high.

Summary and conclusions

1

Cost-benefit studies have been conducted in CMHCs, but these display several methodological problems, such as the use of dubious methods in assigning monetary values to patient improvement (Halpern, 1977), the use of a narrow definition of costs (Levin,1975), the failure to specify whether average or marginal costs are being reported (Murphy & Datel, 1976).

2

Cost-effectiveness studies suffer from similar methodological shortcomings.

3

The measurement of costs should be applied to all resources and inputs, not confined to one 'key' input, nor confined to those inputs which fall within the agency's budget. Costs incurred in other 'constituencies' must be included (see Goldberg & Jones, 1980). The failure to operate this principle is regarded as the main conceptual blockage in studies of efficiency in the mental health field.

4

Technical efficiency has only been studied in one paper (Frank & Taube, 1987) and most of the services studied were free standing out patient clinics, although some CMHCs seem to have been included. Private facilities produced higher outputs than County facilities (with inputs held constant). Decentralised clinics produced 12% more visits than centralised clinics.

5

Some tentative conclusions can be drawn. These are that the costs of maintaining more severely disabled patients tend to be higher; a substantial proportion of the cost savings in community services is due to savings on hospitalisation, and a large proportion of the costs incurred in community services is due to patient hospitalisation (Hafner, 1985). Day services appear to be as effective as DGH services, without being more costly, for certain categories of patient (Dick et al, 1985).

6

The most methodologically sound study (Weisbrod et al, 1980) showed an experimental service to have higher direct treatment costs than a mental hospital, but that all other costs were lower. Patient work productivity was double in the experimental service.

7

When earnings from work are included in cost analyses there is a bias against services with large numbers of retired people, young people, minority groups and those living in areas of high unemployment. Because of their capacity to earn middle class and more educated people return more 'value for money'. Similarly-first admissions return more 'value' than multiple admissions

and voluntary patients return more than involuntary patients.
8
Transferring the lessons of experimental services into 'normal' service provision is fraught with difficulty (Bachrach,1980). Experimental services are able to select subjects, and the costs of providing care for these subjects cannot be generalised to a wider population.
9
The costs of providing care for people with long-term problems is greater than for other groups. People with severe disorders who are cared for in the community require a lot of nursing care, which is expensive (Gudeman et al 1985; Hyde et al, 1987). The cost of providing an effective coordinated service in the community is considerable (Aiken, 1988). Although hostel wards may provide more cost-effective care for these patients when compared with DGH (Teaching) care, they may prove less cost-effective than other forms of care (such as mental hospital care) (Hyde et al, 1987). It is important to make the appropriate cost effectiveness/cost utility comparisons.
10
Different case-mixes produce different cost profiles (May, 1971). Patients who have longer periods in hospital produce greater costs. A method for standardising length of stay, in order to remove the case-mix problem, has been proposed (McMahon, 1985). The major variation in per capita cost is not the length of stay but the admission rate in a community (Taube & Burns, 1988). Service use is not well predicted by diagnosis (Taube et al 1984) or patient characteristics in medical records (Horn et al 1986) but is related to type of hospital and type of clinic (Freiman et al, 1987; Frank & Taube, 1987). Social area characteristics explain the largest amount of the variation in service use (Brandon, 1975; Jencks et al, 1987).
11
The balance of care was not altered by the introduction of CMHCs. The ratio of inpatient to out-patient care remained constant (Brandon, 1975), and the same phenomenon has been observed in the UK (Boardman et al 1987). CMHCs extended care to previously unserved groups, and this could be regarded as an improvement in horizontal target efficiency (Windle et al, 1987); this has also been observed elsewhere (Boardman et al, 1987; Munk-Jorgensen, 1985). The vertical target efficiency of CMHCs, in terms of the proportions of their patients suffering from schizophrenia, for example, was higher (Goldman et al, 1980) than some people supposed (Langsley, 1980).

References

Alessi, L.E. & Wecht, D.J. (1976) The effect of a community mental health center on reducing state hospital admissions. *MD State Med. J.* 65-67.

Bebbington,P., Hurry, J., Tennant, C., Sturt, E., & Wing, J.K. (1981) Epidemiology of mental disorders in Camberwell. *Psychol.Med.* 11(3):561-579.

Binner, P., Halpern, J. & Potter, A. (1973) Patients, programs and results ina comprehensive mental health center. *J.Cons. Clin. Psychol.* 41:148-156.

Boardman, A.P., Bouras, N. & Cundy, J. (1987) *The Mental Health Advice Centre in Lewisham.* London, NUPRD.

Boardman, A.P., Bouras, N. & Watson, J.P. (1986) Evaluation of a community mental health centre. *Acta Psychiat. Belg.* 86:402-406.

Bootman, J.L., Rowland, C., & Wertheimer, A.I. (1979) Cost-benefit analysis. *Evaluation & The Health Professions* 2(2): 129-154.

Bouras, N. & Brough, D.I. (1982) The development of the Mental Health Advice Centre in Lewisham Health District. *Health Trends* 14:65-69.

Brandon, R.N. (1975) Differential use of mental health services: social pathology or class victimization? In Guttentag M. & Struening, E.L. (eds) *Handbook of Evaluation Research.* Beverly Hills, Ca. Sage.

Brown, G. and Craig, T. (1986) Psychiatric cases in community studies: how important an issue? *Soc.Sci.& Med.* 22(2):173-183.

Brown, G.W., Craig, T. & Harris, T.O. (1985) Depression: distress or disease? Some epidemiological considerations. *Brit.J. Psychiat.* 147:612-622.

Challis, D. & Davies, B. (1986) *Case Management in Community Care.* Aldershot, Gower.

Cochran, N. (1979) On the limiting properties of social indicators. *Evaluation & Programme Planning* 2:1-4.

Cooper, B. & Bickel, H. (1984) Population screening and the early detection of dementing disorders in old age: a review. *Psychol.Med.* 14(1):81-9.

DeWitt-Kay, F. (1978) Applications of social area analysis to program planning and evaluation. *J.of eval. & Prog.Planning* 1:65-78.

Dick, P., Cameron, L., Barlow, M. & Ince, A. (1985) Day and Full time Psychiatric Treatment : A Controlled Comparison. *Brit. J. Psychiat.* 147:246-250.

Dickey, B., McGuire, T.G., Cannon, N.L. & Gudeman, J.E. (1986) Mental Health Cost Models: refinements and applications.*Med.Care.* 24:857-867.

Dowell, D.A. & Ciarlo, J.A. (1983) Overview of the Community Mental Health Centers Program from an Evaluation Perspective. *Community Mental Health Journal* 19(2):95-125.

Erdman, H.P., Klein, M.H., Greist, J.H., Bass, S.M., Bires, J.K. & Machtinger, P.E. (1987) A Comparison of the Diagnostic Interview Schedule and Clinical Diagnosis. *Am.J.Psychiat.* 144(1):1477-1480.

Feldstein, M.S. (1984) Econometric studies of health economics. In Intrilligator, M.D. & Kendrick, D.A. *Frontiers of Quantitative Economics*, vol.2. North Holland, Amsterdam.

Fenton, F.R., Tessier, L., Struening, E.L., Smith, F.A., Benoit,C., Contandriopoulas, A.P. & Nguyen, H. (1984) A two year follow-up of a comparative trial of the cost-effectiveness of home and hospital treatment. *Can. J. Psychiat.* 29:205-210.

Finlay-Jones, R.A. & Burvill, P.W. (1977) The prevalence of minor psychiatric morbidity in the community. *Psychol.Med.* 7(3):475-89.

Frank, R. (1981) Cost-Benefit Analysis in Mental Health Services: A Review of the Literature. *Administration in Mental Health* 8(3):161-175.

Frank, R. & Taube, C.A. (1987) Technical and allocative efficiency in the production of out-patient mental health clinic services. *Soc.Sci.Med.* 24(10):843-850.

Freidman, M.P, Mitchell J.B. & Rosenbach, M.L. (1987) An analysis of DRG based reimbursement for Psychiatric Admissions to General Hospitals. *Am. J. Psychiat.* 143:198-200.

Glass, N.J. & Goldberg, D.P. (1977) Cost-benefit analysis and the evaluation of a psychiatric service. *Psychological Med.* 7:701-707.

Goldberg, D.P. (1983) Measurment of the benefits in psychiatry. In Teeling-Smith (ed) *Measuring the Social Benefits of Medicine.* London, HMSO.

Goldberg, D.P. & Jones, R. (1980) The Costs and Benefits of Psychiatric Care. In Robins, L. et al (eds) *The Social Consequences of Psychiatric Illness.* New York, Brunner/Mazel.

Goldberg, D.P. & Huxley, P.J. (1980) *Mental Illness in the Community.* London, Tavistock.

Goldman, H.H., Regier, D.A., Taube, C.A., Redick, R.W. & Bass, R.D. (1980) Community Mental Health Centers and the Treatment of Severe Mental Disorder. *Am.J.Psychiat.* 137 (1): 83-86.

Goodban, N.A., Lieberman, P.B., Levine, M.A., Astrachan, B.M. & Cocilovo, V. (1987) Conceptual and methodological issues in the comparison of inpatient psychiatric facilities. *Am.J.Psychiat.* 144(11):1437-1443.

Goplerud, E., Walfish, S. & Aspey, H. (1983) Surviving cutbacks in community mental health: seventy-seven action strategies. *Community Mental Health Journal* 19:62-76.

Gudeman, J.E., Dickey, B., Evans, A. & Shore, M.F. (1985) Four-year Assessment of a Day Hospital-Inn Program as an Alternative to Inpatient Hospitalisation. *Am.J.Psychiat.* 42(11):1330-1333.

Hafner, H. (1985) Changing Patterns of Mental Health Care. *Acta Psychiatrica Scandinavica* 71, Suppl. 319:151-164.

Hafner, H. & Klug, J. (1982) The impact of an expanding community mental service on patterns of bed usage: evaluation of a four year period of implementation. *Psych.Med.* 12:177-190.

Hagedorn, H.J., Beck, K.J., Neubert, S.F. & Werlin, S.H.(1976) A working manual of simple program evaluation techniques for community mental health centers. *DHEW Publication No. (ADM) 76-404. Rockville, MD. NIMH.*

Hall, G.B. (1988) Monitoring and predicting community mental health centre utilization in Aukland New Zealand. *Soc.Sci.Med.* 26(1):55-70.

Halpern, J. (1977) Program Evaluation, Systems Theory, and Output Value Analysis: A Benefit/Cost Model. In Coursey, R.(ed) *Program Evaluation for Mental Health.* New York, Grune Stratton.

Helzer, J.E., Robins, L.N., McEvoy, L.T. et al (1985) A comparison of clinical and Diagnostic Interview Schedule diagnosis. *Arch. Gen. Psychiat.* 42:656-666.

Herbert, W. (1978) Professional shortfall cited in recent CMHC report. *Am. Psychol. Assoc. Monitor,* Jan.:16-17.

Hodiamont, P., Peer, N. & Syben, N. (1987) Epidemiological aspects of psychiatric disorder in a Dutch health area. *Psychol. Med.* 17(2):495-505.

Horn, S.D., Horn, R.A. & Chambers, R.F. (1986) *Psychiatric Severity of Illness: A Case Mix Study.* Baltimore Center for Hospital Finance & Management, John Hopkins University.

Hutton, F.(1985) Self-referrals to a Community Mental Health Centre: A Three Year Study. *B.J.Psychiat.* 147:540-544.

Huxley, P.J., Korer, J.,Hatfield, B. & Hagan,T. (1987) Evaluating Community Psychiatric Services. *Research Report #2, Mental Health Social Work Research Unit,* Manchester University.

Hyde, C., Bridges, K., Goldberg, D.P., Lowson, K., Sterling, C. & Faragher, B. (1987) The Evaluation of a Hostel Ward: A Controlled Study using Modified Cost-Benefit Analysis. *Brit. J. Psychiat.* 151:805-812.

Jones, K., Sidebotham, R., Wadsworth, W., Tonge, W. & Price, H. (1961) Cost and efficiency in mental hospitals. *The Hospital* 57:23-25.

Jencks, S.F., Horgan, C. & Taube, C. (1987) Bringing excluded psychiatric facilities under the Medicare Prospective Payment System: A Review of Research Evidence and Policy Options. *Medical Care.*

Kane, R.L., Jorgensen, L.A.B. & Pepper, G.A. (1974) Can nursing home care be cost-effective? *J.Am.Geriat.Soc.* 22:265-272.

Kane, R.L., Jorgensen, L.A., Teteberg, B. & Kuwahara, J. (1976) Is good nursing home care feasible? *JAMA* 235(5):516-519.

Katon, W. (1986) Panic disorder: epidemiology, diagnosis, and treatment in primary care. *J.Clin.Psychiat.* 47,Suppl.P,21-30

Katon, W. (1987) The epidemiology of depression in medical care. *Int.J.Psychiatry Med.* 17(1):93-112.

Keisler, C.A. (1982) Public and professional myths about mental hospitalisation: an empirical reassessment of policy related beliefs. *Am. Psychol.* 37:1323-1329.

Knapp, M. (1984) *The economics of social care.* London, Macmillan.

Langsley, D.G. (1980) The Community Mental Health Center: Does it treat patients? *Hosp. & Community Psychiatry* 31(12):815-819.

Leaf, P.J., Bruce, M.L. & Tischler, G.L. (1986) The differential effect of attitudes on the use of mental health services.*Soc. Psychiat.* 21:187-192.

Lehman, A.F., Babigian, H.M. & Reed, S.K. (1984) The epidemiology of treatment for chronic and nonchronic mental disorders. *J.Nerv.Ment.Dis.* 172(11):658-666.

Levin, H. (1975) Cost-effectiveness analysis in evaluation research. In Guttentag M. & Struening, E.L. (eds) *Handbook of Evaluation Research.* Beverly Hills, Ca. Sage.

Levine, S. (1987) The changing terrains of medical sociology: emergent concern with Quality of Life. *J.Health Soc. Behav.* 28(1):1-6.

Luft, L.L. & Fakhouri, J. (1979) A Model for a Comparative Cost-effectiveness Evaluation of Two Mental Health Partial Care Programs. *Evaluation and Program Planning*, 2:33-40.

Marks, I. Connolly, J. & Muijen, M. (eds) *New Directions in Mental Health Care Evaluation.* Institute of Psychiatry, London.

May, P. (1970) Cost-effectiveness of mental health care, Part II. *Am.J.Pub.Health* 60(12):2269-2272.

May, P. (1971) Cost-efficiency of mental health delivery systems. *Am.J.Pub. Health* 60(11):2060-2067.

McGuire, T.G. & Fairbank, A. (1988) Patterns of mental health utilisation over time in a fee for service population. *Am.J.Pub.Health* 78(2):134-136.

McMahon, S.M. (1985) The Efficiency of Inpatient Medical Care in a Hospital Secure Unit. *Med.Care* 23(10):1139-1147.

Miller, G.H., Dear, M. & Streiner, D.L. (1986) A model for predicting utilisation of psychiatric facilities. *Can. J. Psychiat.* 31:424-430.

Munk-Jorgensen, P. (1985) Cumulated need for psychiatric service as shown in the community psychiatric project. *Psychol. Med.* 15:629-635.

Murphy, J.G. & Datel, W.E. (1976) A cost-benefit analysis of community versus institutional living. *Hosp.& Comm.Psychia try* 27(3):165-170.

Mustian, R.D. & See, J.J. (1973) Indicators of mental health needs: an empirical and pragmentic evaluation. *J.Health & Soc. Behav.* 14:23-28.

NIMH (1977) *Community Mental Health Centers: the federal investment.* Rockville, MD.

Ochberg, F.M. (1976) Community mental health centre legislation: flight of the phoenix. *Am.J.Psychiat.* 133(1):56-61.

Pardes, H. & Stockdill, J.W. (1984) Survival Strategies for Community Mental Health Services in the 1980s. *Hospital & Community Psychiatry* 35(2):127-132.

Peet, M. (1986) Network Community Mental Health Care in North-West Derbyshire. *Bulletin of the Royal College of Psychiatrists* 10:262-265.

Potter, A., Binner, P. & Halpern, J. (1975) Readmission discount factors in program evaluation. *Am.J.Comm.Psychol.* 3:305-314.

Reich, J. (1986) The epidemiology of anxiety. *J.Ner.Ment.Dis.* 174 (3):129-136.

Reynolds, I, Rizzo, C. & Gallagher, H. (1981) The prevalence of psychosocial problems. A study of 37,678 Sydney adults. *Aust. Fam. Physician.* 10(9):734-738.

Robins, L. N., Helzer, J.E., Ratcliff, K.F. et al (1982) Validity of the Diagnostic Interview Schedule, Version II: DSM-III diagnoses. *Psychol. Med.* 12:855-870.

Rothenberg, J. (1975) Cost-benefit analysis: A Methodological Exposition. In Guttentag M. & Struening, E.L. (eds) *Handbook of Evaluation Research.* Beverly Hills, Ca. Sage.

Sackett, D.L. & Holland, W.W. (1975) Controversy in the detection of disease. *Lancet* ii:357-359.

Schaeffer, D.E., Schulberg, H.C. & Board, G. (1978) Effects of Community Mental Health Services on Stat Hospital Admissions: A Clinical-Demographic study. *Hosp. & Community Psych.* 29(9):579-583.

Scheffler, R. & Rossiter, L.(eds) (1983) *Advances in Health Economics and Health Services Research.* JAI Press, Greenwich, Conn.

Shapiro, S., Skinner, E.A., Kessler, L.G., Von-Korff, M., German, P.S., Tischler, G.L., Leaf, P.J., Benham, L., Cottler, L., & Regier, D. (1984) Utilization of health and mental health services. Three Epidemiologic Catchment Area sites. *Arch. Gen.Psychiat.* 41(10):971-978.

Sharfstein, S. (1978) Will Community Mental Health Survive in the 1980s? *Am. J.Psychiat.* 135(11):1363-1365.

Sharfstein, S. & Clark, H. (1978) Economics and the chronic mental patient. *Schizophrenia Bulletin* 4:399-414.

Sharfstein, S. & Nafziser, J.C. (1976) Community Care: costs and benefits for a chronic patient. *Hospital and Community Psychiatry* 27:170-173.

Struening, E.L. (1983) Social Area Analysis as a method of evaluation. In Struening E.L. (ed) *Handbook of evaluation research.* New York, Sage.

Taube, C.A. & Burns, B. J. (1988) Cross-national evaluations of mental health services delivery and financing: some collaboration opportunities. In Marks, I. Connolly, J. & Muijen, M. (eds) *New Directions in Mental Health Care Evaluation.* Institute of Psychiatry, London.

Taube, C., Lee, E.S. & Forthofer, R. (1984) DRGs in Psychiatry: An empirical evaluation. *Medical Care* 22:597-610.

Wadsworth, W., Tonge, W. & Barber, L. (1957) The cost and efficiency of mental hospitals. *Lancet* 2:533-534.

Warheit, G.J., Buhl, J.M. & Bell, R.A. (1978) A critique of social indicators analysis and key informants surveys as needs assessment methods. *Evaluation and Program Planning* 1:239-247.

Weisbrod, B.A., Test, M.A., & Stein, L.I.(1980) Alternative to Mental Hospital treatment: Economic Benefit-Cost Analysis. *Arch. Gen. Psychiat.* 37:400-405.

Weissman, M.M. (1987) Advances in psychiatric epidemiology: rates and risks for major depression. *A.J.Pub.Health* 77(4): 445-51.

Wells, K.B., Hough, R.L., Golding, J.M., Burnam, M. & Karno M. (1987) Which Mexican-Americans underutilize health services? *Am. J.Psychiat.* 144(7):918-922.

Williams, A. & Anderson, R.(1975) *Efficiency in the Social Services.* Oxford, Blackwell.

Williams, A. (1977) Measuring the Quality of Life. In Wingo, L. & Evans, A. (eds) *Public Economics and The Quality of Life.* The John Hopkins University Press.

Williams, D.H. (1986) The epidemiology of mental illness in Afro-Americans. *Hosp.Community Psychiat.* 37(1):42-49.

Williams, P. (1986) Mental Illness and Primary Care: Screening. In Shepherd,M., Wilkinson, G. & Williams, P. (eds) *Mental Illness in Primary Care Settings.* London, Tavistock.

Windle, C., Bass, R.D. & Gray, L. (1987) The impact of federally funded CMHCs on local mental health service systems. *Hosp.Comm. Psychiat.* 38(7):729-734.

Windle, C. & Scully, D.(1976) Community Mental Health Centers and the Decreasing Use of State Mental Hospitals. *Community Mental Health Journal* 12(3):239-243.

Wing, J.K. & Hailey, A.M.(1972) *Evaluating a Community Psychiatric Service.* London, O.U.P.

Winslow, W.W. (1982) Changing Trends in CMHCs: Keys to Survival in the Eighties. *Hosp. & Community Psychiat.* 33(4):273-277.

Woof, K., Freeman, H.L. & Fryers, T. (1983) Psychiatric service use in Salford. A comparison of point-prevalence ratios in 1968 and 1978. *Brit.J.Psychiat.* 142:588-597.

Woy, J.R., Wasserman, D.B. & Weiner-Pomerantz, R. (1981) Community mental health centers: movement away from the model? *Community Mental Health Journal* 17(4):265-276.

Yates, W.R. (1986) The NIMH epidemiologic study: implications for family practice. *J.Fam.Pract.* 22(3):251-255.

5 Effective services

Introduction

This chapter is concerned with those studies which attempt to assess the effectiveness of CMHCs. We have decided to concentrate on studies which assess the outcome of intervention rather than on studies which judge service performance in relation to service objectives. We feel that the latter are more a matter for the consideration of service managers, are of less relevance than direct assessments of patient/client outcomes, and are more prone to problems of definition and hence problems of validity and reliability. We do look at these issues briefly in the chapter on evaluation. Another important reason for concentrating on outcomes rather than the structures and processes of services is that there has been a major shift of emphasis in relation to the community care of mentally ill people in the UK. The white paper 'Caring for People' makes it clear that, in future, the actual outcome of the service provided will be the focus of attention. The view of the service user will need to be taken into account, and where local social services authorities become the purchasers of care rather than the providers they will, in turn, be interested in whether the contracted out services which they purchase are provided effectively and efficiently. It is hard to see how they will do this without assessing the outcome for the service users.

Important aspects of service performance in relation to target groups have been examined in the chapter on efficiency, but some of the same studies are reviewed again here, when they present well-substantiated and relevant findings. With one or two exceptions, we are only interested in studies which produce outcome data relating to individual clients. For the most part we will not be concerned with studies of effectiveness in relation to hidden morbidity or prevention. We will concentrate on identified morbidity.

Reviews of effectiveness

In their review of the performance of CMHCs, Howell and Ciarlo (1983) summarise the achievements of CMHC's. Using seven goals derived from the enabling legislation (P.L. 88 - 164, Title II) and associated regulations, they examine CMHC performance. On the basis of the evidence which they review they draw the following conclusions:

> The CMHC program's major achievement has been to increase the range and quantity of public mental health services.
> For some poor and minority groups services became more available and accessible.
> In some urban areas services were provided to meet existing community needs, but some clinical target group and rural area needs were not met.

They note that the attainment of these goals by community based services became increasingly difficult after the withdrawal of federal support, although Woy et al (1981) argued that this tendency could be observed before federal funding ceased. After federal funding ceased there was a move away from the comprehensive mixture of community based services towards hospital based care, especially inpatient care. They attribute this shift to the reimbursement criteria of public and private insurers which favour services used by the most severely disturbed patients. This increases, rather than decreases, costs because out-patient and partial hospitalisation services are cheaper.

We have seen in the efficiency Chapter that after federal funding ended, many centres had fiscal problems and had to develop strategies to cope with financial cut-backs. Many of these strategies involved earning more, by concentrating on the more lucrative hospital services. Thompson et al (1982), on the basis of NIMH and Census Bureau data, observe that the period of the growth of CMHCs coincided with broader access to services, and increasing use of out-patient and community based services. Latterly however they detect increasing reliance on private care with the help of third-party reimbursement.

There is a possibility that something similar may happen in the UK, unless private insurance is introduced which provides cover for community services at the same, or preferably an advantageous rate, compared with private cover for hospital care. If mental illness services for long-term and severely disabled patients are to be coordinated in the community by social agencies, while 'health care' is provided by the hospitals, then it is clear that the bulk of health insurance funds will go to private 'hospital', and not private 'community', or public 'community' care.

Effectiveness studies in CMHCs

Dowell and Ciarlo suggest that the appropriate effectiveness measures to use, in any service comparisons, are the impact upon client functioning, the burden and benefits to family, and service utilisation and recidivism. We have examined service utilisation, and cost-benefit and cost-effectiveness studies in the chapter on efficiency, so we will confine the present review of effectiveness to the other aspects.

We have structured the literature in the following way, around studies of:

clinical/ social outcome effectiveness reported from CMHCs
outcome in terms of readmission
outcome of consultation and education
the use of goal-attainment scaling
the outcome for patients with long-term problems, with particular reference to aftercare programmes

Clinical and social outcome

The two goals of 'efficiency' and 'effectiveness' were not added to the CMHC program until 1977. Dowell and Ciarlo observe that efficiency is hard to assess, and conclude that in some areas, such as the co-ordination of aftercare services in the community the CMHCs have not been successful. They are unable to draw any firm conclusion at all about effectiveness, due to the limited number of well-designed evaluative studies.

We can confirm that the number of studies of the effectiveness of CMHCs remains limited. There are many more papers concerned with proposals and schemes for evaluation, but which provide no data which test the proposals. A brief review of the range of methodological issues discussed in these papers is given in a later chapter. Because of the limited number of rigorous studies of CMHCs, we have extended the review to consider those studies of services which most closely resemble CMHCs in design or intention. This leads us to include studies which describe services which have been established with the same aims and basic structure as CMHCs, (see Dowell & Ciarlo, 1983) but to exclude studies which consider the effectiveness of treatment in hospital, i.e. inpatient and out-patient services, or day hospitals (e.g Wilkinson, 1984; Tyrer, 1987); (except where these are compared with community alternatives, or involve the assessment of costs). We have excluded studies which refer specifically to the reprovision of services for the 'old long stay' patients, and to rehabilitation services based in hospital (e.g. Paul & Lentz,1977; Lavender,1987).

We do not pretend that this is always an easy distinction to maintain. For instance, we note that the definition of 'deinstitutionalisation' used by NIMH in the USA, includes the prevention of admission through the use of community alternatives, and aftercare services for noninstitutionalised people receiving community services (Bachrach, 1977). In other words, pretty well everything!

Dowell and Ciarlo resort to using evidence from psychotherapy outcome research to try to substantiate the effectiveness of CMHCs. Success by implication is not evidence of effectiveness. Studies which show the increased effectiveness of partial care or brief hospitalisation are more relevant; they show the advantages of reduced dependence upon long periods of hospital inpatient care for most groups of patients (viz Dick et al, 1985; Falloon & Talbot, 1982; Herz et al, 1975; Riessman et al , 1977; Washburn et al, 1976).

Tantam (1985) reviews this literature and feels that we can safely draw the following conclusions about the performance of community based alternatives to mental hospitals:

That satisfaction with community based programmes is greater than with conventional brief admission and aftercare (Stein & Test, 1980; Hoult & Reynolds, 1984).

The best results are found in comparisons with custodial state mental hospital treatment (Pasamanick et al, 1964); in the use of partial hospital care for patients with families (Hertz et al,1975), and for selected patients in a residential therapeutic community (Mosher et al, 1975).

That in all experimental programmes many community residents have to be readmitted to hospital.

That it is reasonable to assume that cost-effective treatment methods in the USA are likely to prove so in the UK, but that the divided responsibility for service provision in the UK slows progress towards a unified services, and that more attention has been paid, particularly by psychiatrists, to improving hospital rather than community care.

Conventional aftercare could be improved, and questions need to be asked about the most effective redeployment of hospital staff in community settings, as well as about the specific 'therapeutic ingredients' of community provisions.

While psychiatric practice in the two countries differs,(for instance there is a greater reliance on the use of hospitalisation in the USA), the need for hospital admission for some patients, at certain points in their illness, remains a necessary and useful component in a wide range of service provision. The fact that it continues to be the best funded part of service provision is not, in Tantam's view, due to 'mere prejudice' on the part of psychiatrists.

The weight of evidence is certainly on the side of the effectiveness of community services, with certain limitations. An increasingly significant limitation is that much of the evidence for the efficacy of community services comes from well-funded **experimental** alternatives, and conventional services require considerable improvement in order to perform as effectively. Co-ordination of service provisions involving several different agencies, can be particularly difficult to manage in the community. Braun et al (1981) reach the same conclusions after an extensive review of the literature on deinstitutionalisation (based on the wide definition of this term referred to above). The ability of so-called 'model' programs to generalise to conventional services has been questioned. Bachrach (1980) cites the obstacles to generalisation (see Evaluation chapter).

A further conclusion which can be drawn from the evidence to date is that social factors have a significant bearing on the onset, course and outcome of minor and major psychiatric disorders. Studies which predict outcome, consistently show social factors to perform as well as, and usually better than clinical factors (Huxley et al,1979; Mann et al, 1981; Sartorius, 1977; Strauss & Carpenter, 1974; Wittenborn et al, 1977). Diagnosis and clinical symptomatology at the onset of the disorder are not good predictors of outcome. As we have seen above (efficiency chapter) and below (evaluation chapter) social factors are also predictive of service utilisation, whereas diagnosis, and diagnostic related groups are fairly weak predictors. The well known work on the onset of depression in women (Brown & Harris, (1978), and on relapse and family interventions in schizophrenia (Barrowclough & Tarrier, 1984; Strachan, 1986) shows that the assessment, and effective care and treatment of people with mental disorder, owes a great deal to the successful integration of a social perspective. The importance of social factors should be reflected in the processes of the development and implementation of social policy. Without the integration of health and social perspectives the service for clients simply cannot hope to be effective.

Readmission as outcome

Readmission rates to mental health facilities have often been used as indicators of treatment effectiveness (Anthony et al, 1972; Franklin et al, 1975; Turner et al, 1979).

The rate of readmissions reported in the literature remains

fairly constant, at 35-45%. Turner, however, has pointed out that the use of readmission rates as indicators of the outcome of treatment is so fraught with difficulty as to be almost useless, while others observe that follow-up studies lack comparability in basic respects (Bachrach, 1976).

A reasonable case can be made for readmissions to be considered an indicator of treatment success rather than failure. This is particularly true in respect of community based treatment agencies when they are aiming to serve people with long-term, or recurrent disorders, who may need early intervention, but who, in the past, have been reluctant to seek help.

In order to be meaningful readmissions statistics should distinguish between readmission for the same problem as last time, and readmission for a new problem. This is often not reported. Turner also point out that readmissions are a function of the size and age of an agency or centre, and that comparing two centres of a different age is likely only to confirm their age as a major determinant of readmission rate (Rutlege & Binner,1970).

The accuracy of data collected about readmissions leaves a good deal to be desired. There are many different definitions in use: some cases are counted as readmissions only when services are offered, whereas others represent 'head counts' of everyone who presents at reception. In some cases whole families are counted as one case, while in others each individual member is counted as a case. The type of problem is sometimes not recorded, or not reported. When this happens it is not possible to take into account the fact that the problem may be an entirely new episode of something for which the client has never received treatment before.

Other important considerations are: the age of the client at successive admissions; the time between the admission and readmission; the treatment environment to which the client returns (is it the same as the previous one, or could it be said to be a readmission to a less restrictive facility, i.e. out-patient rather than inpatient status); and how to account for multiple readmissions in the system of recording.

In some studies, index and control groups are compared up to the time at which readmission takes place. Readmitted and non-readmitted groups are then studied, and, frequently, attempts are made to predict readmission status, from a host of other variables. If the readmission is not seen as a failure, but rather as part of the treatment programme, then it is possible for readmitted cases to benefit from the period of treatment be discharged, and have a better outcome at a fixed follow-up point, than clients who remain in the community, but who may be in a deteriorating condition. These studies assume that community tenure is synonymous with a 'good' outcome, or treatment success, and readmitted patients are synonymous with treatment failure (e.g Kirk 1976). Without a follow-up assessment, at a fixed point, of cases in the community one cannot be certain that this is the case. There is a near uniform tendency to assume that hospital stay consists of a smooth path to recovery, and to ignore the fact that (depending on length of stay) a patient may relapse once, or more often, while still in hospital.

These, and the other limitations of readmission measures, reduce their value as indicators of effectiveness, and as indicators of service performance. Problems with measurement and design may also account for two of the common findings of studies based on readmission rates. These two findings are: that aftercare does not affect readmission and that social factors do not distinguish between readmitted and non-readmitted groups (Solomon et al, 1984). A comparison between readmitted cases, at the point of readmission, and others not readmitted, using data from the index admission, will not capture the true range of outcome possibilities. Cases in the community may have better, or worse clinical and social outcomes than the readmitted cases. In addition, there is immense variation in the nature of readmission itself. The reasons for readmission may be associated with: severe clinical relapse or prevention of clinical deterioration; with an episode of a new disorder or an 'old' disorder; and with problems with or without social precipitants. In these circumstances it is perhaps not surprising that variables collected at an index admission, whether clinical or social, are unable to predict readmission status accurately (e.g. Wessler & Iven, 1970).

Finally, studies which compare outcome of one group in terms of readmission, with the outcome of another which has not been readmitted at the time of follow-up, could be said to be studying 'time to readmission'. Unfortunately this study design does not allow the second group to reach the point of readmission.

The major conclusions which are repeated in the literature are as follows. People who are evaluated at a CMHC are less likely to be hospitalised than those assessed at a mental hospital. This is usually because the mental hospitals have access to fewer, or no, alternatives to hospitalisation than the CMHC. If they are hospitalised, they spend fewer days as inpatients and are less frequently readmitted (Dyck, 1974; Sheridan & Teplin, 1981; Stubblebine & Decker, 1971).

The most consistent finding is that patients who have been admitted once will have a high frequency of admissions (Freeman & Simmons, 1963; Burvill & Mittleman, 1971; Rosenblatt & Mayer, 1974; Fontana & Dowds, 1975; Kirk, 1976; Sheridan & Teplin, 1981). Sheridan & Teplin (1981) point out that readmission can be due not only to exacerbation of the severity of the symptoms, but also to: expectations of rehospitalization by the ex-patient, relatives and friends; greater stress as a result of the stigma which arises in the community in respect of former patients; a bias among professionals towards previously hospitalised patients; and a tendency to use hospital services, rather than alternatives.

Sheridan & Teplin (1981) compared the readmission rates of patients originally referred by the police to CMHCs and state hospital. Geographical sectors determined whether the patient went to CMHC or hospital. The two groups of patients did not differ in terms of sociodemography except that a greater proportion of ethnic minority patients were admitted to the state hospital (an artifact of the demography of the catchment area). Approximately three-quarters of both groups had previous hospitalisations.

Fifty-six per cent of those seen at the CMHC were hospitalised compared to 79% seen at the state hospital. The proportions referred for out-patient care were 29% at the CMHC, and 9% at the state hospital. Readmissions of the state hospital group were significantly higher at both 1 and 2 year follow-up. Patients, on average, spent fifty days in the state hospital but nineteen days in the CMHC.

This group of patients represented some of the most difficult to treat; they were usually acutely disturbed; frequently diagnosed a suffering from schizophrenia; often lacking insight; unable to care for themselves; and often suicidal or homicidal. The study confirms that, even in an alternative system, a large number of these patient do require hospitalisation, albeit for short periods in some cases. In terms of rehospitalization only, this study confirms that outcome is better for CMHC patients than state hospital patients. The use of fixed follow-up periods avoids some of the methodological problems referred to above. However, the quality of outcome was not studied, and the comparison might be more meaningful if another service was used, rather than the state hospital, which has very few options other than to admit.

Aftercare services

We tend to concur with Hoult (1986) who says that the term 'aftercare' carries the unfortunate connotation that what happens in aftercare, comes 'after' the main, and most important treatment as already taken place. In fact, the literature is unanimous on one thing: successful services rely less upon hospital care, and more upon the provision of adequate and coordinated community care. This conclusion applies to all patients who are admitted to hospital (Goering et al, 1984; Gloag, 1985), patients with long term problems (Test,1981; Wilkinson, 1985), and deinstitutionalisation programmes (Braun et al, 1981) including the Italian experience (Tansella & Williams, 1987). Successful services work out the proper place for hospital care, and do not regard the community services and the hospital services as polar opposites (Tantam, 1985).

Tansella et al (1987) found that, as in most other countries, expenditure on Italian hospital services still far outweighed the expenditure on community services. This was almost ten years after the introduction of Law 180, which was aimed at the creation of a comprehensive and integrated system of community care. The CENSIS survey (1984) found a tenfold variation (between the regions with the best and the worst provision) in the provision of catchment based community psychiatric services and facilities.

Test (1981) reviews the evidence for chronic patients. She concludes that aftercare services, to be effective for this group of patients should: be based on individualised care plans; be 'assertive' i.e. going to clients to help them, rather than expecting them to come to the services; provide care continuously, possibly through a case-management system (Ozarin,1978; Challis & Davies, 1986; Whitehead, 1987; Huxley, 1990); not be time limited. Hoult (1986), not surprisingly reached very similar conclusions in a replication of Stein & Test's work, in Australia.

Test notes that when an aftercare programme ceases, patient gains are reversed. This has been known for a long time with regard to drug treatments, but is also true of community based therapy programmes (Langsley et al, 1971; Stein & Test, 1980) and of special employment programmes (Fairweather, 1969)

Solomon et al (1980) investigated a continuing care programme for discharged severely ill patients in California. The patients were mostly schizophrenia sufferers (70%) and most had been hospitalised at least twice during the previous twelve months. 263 referrals were made to the service during 18 months. The service consisted of three multidisciplinary teams, emphasising outreach, with most members of the team out in the field most of the time. At referral 121 patients were in locked facilities, 61 in boarding out, and 38 in independent settings. At 18 months the number in locked facilities dropped to 86, and the number in independent living rose to 82.

Although hospital admissions were reduced by one third during the same period, a small number of patients still required frequent admissions. In addition, 119 patients were engaged in little or no activity. 60% of those in boarding out were engaged in 'meaningful activities', but 60% of those living independently did nothing. 20% of the independent living group were engaged in open employment or sheltered work. The authors note that, 'helping this population to engage in more meaningful activities was a harder task than expected. The verbal emphasis in day treatment was inappropriate for many clients, Therapists' expectations about vocational rehabilitation were often too high, and jobs in any case were scarce....it was difficult to get the staff to accept the concept of limited goals or the idea that the prevention of backward movement represented success.' These findings echo those referred to by Brown (1973) in his description of the problems facing mental hospital staff.

The pattern of aftercare in the community has been described in three studies which each included over 500 patients (Kirk, 1976; Solomon et al, 1983; and Goering et al, 1984). Unfortunately both the studies by Kirk and Solomon et al only followed up patients until they were readmitted (see above). Goering et al used fixed follow-up points, and is therefore more satisfactory. The other two studies are nevertheless instructive in what they tell us about the type and amount of aftercare provided before readmission.

Kirk (1976) using computerised data files and records from mental hospital and community services obtained information on the 579 people discharged from hospital during a twelve month period, and for a three year period following index hospitalisation. 56% had at least one contact with a CMHC between leaving hospital, and readmission, or the end of the three years. 55% received some form of after care service from the CMHC, and of these half were seen on seven occasions or less, and 90% were seen on less than 53 days. The total hours of service ranged from 1 to 1000, with a median of 6.1. A few patients did not receive aftercare until more than one year after discharge (7%); 30% received it within a week and 65% within a month.

Bearing in mind the methodological problems in this study, it is nevertheless interesting to note that a higher proportion of patients in receipt of aftercare were readmitted (41%) than those not in receipt (31%). Many of those not in receipt of service, and not readmitted were well, but the nonreadmitted group included those who received more than eleven days of service. Those who received some, but not much aftercare were the ones who were readmitted. Kirk shows that aftercare services were more often offered to patients with high levels of chronicity, but that the amount of service was not related to chronicity level. The higher the chronicity score the more likely was the patient to be readmitted.

Solomon et al (1983) tracked a cohort of 550 patients through a mental health after care service, and included data on the patients reported by other agencies. Follow-up was after one year or at the point of readmission. 60% had a diagnosis of schizophrenia, 83% had one or more previous admissions. The authors report that most patients did connect with the aftercare services (66%), and when they included the admitted patients time to follow-up this rose to 75%. When the welfare agencies were included 82 % made contact. 48% made contact within a week and 79% within a month. The mean time in care was 194 days. The median time of service received was 12 hours. The median number of hours of individual therapy was 5.5. Social rehabilitation median hours was 2.5, and the mean 20 hours.

Solomon et al conclude that the services are primarily maintenance oriented, rather than rehabilitative. The levels of service provided are very low. The authors do not give any indication of the appropriateness of the services offered, nor their outcome. It is hard to draw any further conclusions, other than that the level of provision, given the nature of the handicaps involved, seems inadequate.

Goering et al (1984) describe 6 month and 2 year outcomes for 505 subjects, in a traditional system of service delivery in Toronto. The hospital included a research institute, two general hospitals and a provincial hospital. 35% of the subjects were suffering from schizophrenia and 25% from other psychoses, and 21% from personality disorder or alcoholism. 29% had had six or more previous admissions, and 50% had had between one and five admissions.

One third were readmitted within six months, and two-thirds within 2 years. Those with fewer previous admissions were less likely to be readmitted. At six months more than half were withdrawn, and one third expressed hostility or suspiciousness. 40% were dissatisfied with their living conditions, and the research confirmed that 20% did live in inadequate conditions. Subjects reported that loneliness and boredom were their biggest problems. 45% of subjects had no contact with aftercare services during the first 6 months. Because of the non-experimental nature of the design, i.e. normal services were allowed to operate, there was very little evidence of discharge planning with regard to aftercare.

These three studies show that aftercare varies enormously, often does not reach the patient very quickly, and seems to be unplanned and haphazard. We have very little evidence from normally operating services, that there is much pre-discharge planning, and little evidence that appropriate aftercare reaches those in most need of it. Apart from some experimental programmes already referred to, there is little evidence of the effectiveness of 'normal' aftercare services.

Hammaker (1983) studied the impact on state hospital use, of a statewide implementation of community support services. People with a severe disorder and impaired role functioning were provided with a new service requiring a range of community support provisions, including case management, outreach, daily support, vocational skill development, and residential resource development. Hospital data for the five years preceding the service, and for one year's operation of the new service were compared for 400 randomly selected service users.

Rehospitalization rates and lengths of hospital stay declined when the new service was introduced. Unfortunately the data are not tested for statistical significance, and some of the comparisons with other services included some inappropriate groups (e.g childrens' services).

It should come as no surprise to learn that the more problems patients experience on return to the community, the more likely they are to want to return to the hospital. In a twelve month follow-up study of 176 patients discharged from mental hospitals in Massachusetts, Kinard (1981) found that one quarter said that they had wanted to return to the hospital at some time during the year after discharge. Of those who said that they had wanted to return, 58% were feeling depressed, 36% wanted asylum, 22% missed their friends at the hospital, and 18% preferred the controlled environment of the hospital. Decreased participation in social activities after discharge was associated with wanting to return.

The results of this study are instructive but cannot be definitive because of the high attrition rate in the sample. 583 patients were discharged, but only 176 interviewed. Those lost to the study did not differ in socio-demographic characteristics or previous history, length of stay and diagnosis. The respondents were more likely to have a drug prescribed at discharge.

The findings are similar to those of a small study of discharged patients attending for psychiatric treatment (modecate injection) at an inner city health centre in the UK (Huxley, 1986). A number of these patients, although maintained in the community were socially isolated and living in inadequate housing. Few of the patients were in contact with aftercare services, and those that were often reported them as unsuitable, or unavailable. One patient described returning to the hospital for social contacts, and for some patients the trip to the clinic was their only excursion out of their homes.

It is unfortunate that more systematic study of after care has not been undertaken. There is now considerable but not conclusive evidence that the long term outcome for schizophrenia in particular, is not as gloomy as has been thought. It seems possible that well organised after care services might play a crucial part in the course of schizophrenic illness. We think that it is worthwhile reviewing the evidence here, not least because it lends weight to the argument, regularly expressed by British health ministers at the present time, that patients should not be discharged from hospital before adequate services are available in the community.

Harding et al (1987a) report that each of the five long term follow up studies reported since 1972 all shown similar results for the course of schizophrenic illness. Half or more of the patients in each study had significantly improved or recovered at 20, 30 or 40 year follow up. Bleuler (1968) followed up 208 patients first admitted during 1942 and 1943. 23% of the first admissions achieved full recovery and an additional 43% sustained significant improvement. In 1965 Deane and Brooks (Deane & Brooks, 1967) followed up a cohort of 269 patients from the back wards of Vermont state hospital. When they were admitted to the study these patients had been ill for an average of 16 years, totally disabled for 10, and hospitalised continuously for 6. At follow up they found that two thirds could be maintained in the community if sufficient transitional facilities and adequate aftercare were provided. When followed up again in the 1980's (Harding et al, 1987) 34% of those diagnosed schizophrenic were fully recovered in both psychiatric and social terms. An additional 34% were significantly improved.

Similar results have been obtained elsewhere, in both rural and urban communities. For instance the recovery rate in Lausanne was 29% (Ciompi & Muller, 1976), in Bonn 26% (and 31% significantly improved)(Huber et al, 1979) and in Iowa (Tsuang et al, 1979) 20% (26% significantly improved).

Harding et al (1987b) report that the outcome for half to two thirds of the schizophrenia sufferers was 'neither downward nor marginal' but 'an evolution into various degrees of productivity, social involvement, wellness and competent functioning'. It is not clear form this study or the others, what contribution aftercare makes to the outcome, but Harding makes the point that after care services were already in place before the patients left the hospital in Vermont. This lends weight to the argument that after care is probably important, and might make a central contribution to the course of disorder, when organised properly. The cynic might suggest that in the UK, the tendency to be pessimistic about the outcome of major mental illness could conceivably have been fuelled by the woefully inadequate record of local authority after care provision over the last thirty years.

Burden on the families of patients

A large and well known literature has emerged over the last twenty years on the extent to which psychiatric patients appear to be responsible for psychological, social and economic burdens on their families. It would not be appropriate to review all this work in detail, but in summary we can say that the research has shown that the effects on others is an important dimension in the measurement of treatment effectiveness.

Studies have shown that relatives bear an often unacknowledged burden of care (Creer & Wing, 1974; Lamb & Oliphant, 1978), and suffer disrupted family life, and considerable personal distress (Grad & Sainsbury, 1963; Test & Stein, 1980; Hughes, 1978). Most relatives feel 'subjective' burden (Gillis & Keet, 1965; Wing et al,1964), especially in relation to psychotic symptoms (Brown, 1959; Hughes, 1978). A significant number, however, perhaps as many as 40%, do not report subjective burden in the face of objective problems (Brown, 1958; Gillis & Keet, 1965; Hoenig & Hamilton, 1969). Hoenig & Hamilton (1969) call this discrepancy 'tolerance'. Greenley (1979) suggests that family tolerance of symptomatic behaviour is the key factor in preventing rehospitalization. He identified similar levels of symptomatic behaviour in groups of rehospitalized and nonrehospitalized patients, and argued that family tolerance levels were higher in the nonrehospitalized group. He also found that families were most uneasy in the face of psychotic behaviour, more so than in the face of overtly dangerous behaviour. The study was based on a small sample, due to a high attrition rate, but the results tend to confirm those of earlier work.

Without the family care of psychiatric patients, services would be overwhelmed. The same is true of service for other groups of people with handicaps and dependency needs (Bayley, 1973; Greengross, 1982; Wenger, 1984). Non-statutory care is essential to the maintenance of community care in general (Moroney, 1976), and the community care of mentally ill people in particular (Hatfield, 1978). There are good reasons to suppose that the informal care networks which operate to maintain elderly people in the community, may be absent or deficient in respect of mentally ill people, placing an even greater burden on families (Huxley, 1990). 'Tolerance' may be a function of the relatives past failure to mobilise help from informal sources (and formal sources), leading to a feeling of resignation.

Families who have received a family management approach rather than an individual or patient oriented approach, report less disruption of activities, and less subjective burden (Falloon & Pederson, 1985). Following the pioneering work of Brown et al (1972), both Vaughn & Leff (1976) and later Falloon and his colleagues (1985) developed methods for the identification of 'expressed emotion' in the families of schizophrenia sufferers, and therapeutic approaches aimed at the reduction of the stress induced by high levels of expressed emotion. These methods are, broadly speaking, family approaches to problem solving, involving education about schizophrenia.

The support and information given to relatives had a powerful effect on relatives ability to cope, in a study in Australia (Hoult,1986; Reynolds & Hoult, 1984). Reynolds & Hoult compared a community based approach, (based on Stein & Test's work) with standard psychiatric care. Patients were randomly allocated to the two services. As well as demonstrating a better outcome for the community service, in terms of hospitalisation, treatment costs, and clinical outcome, nearly all the relatives preferred the community treatment. The control group's relatives complained that help was not available when it was needed, home visits by staff were rare, and staff showed little interest in and spent little time with patients. The authors add a sensible cautionary note, (referred to above), to the effect that the service may not be as effective when it ceases to be 'experimental' and becomes part of the normal pattern of service provision.

Goal attainment scaling

The evaluation of client improvement has been undertaken using the Goal Attainment Scaling (GAS) system (Kiresuk & Sherman, 1968; Kiresuk & Lund, 1975). Calsyn & Davidson (1978) report the 'GAS in some form or another has been adopted in hundreds of human service agencies'.

In view of the extensive use of this system, it is appropriate to include a brief description here, but we share with Calsyn & Davidson (1979) and Cytrynbaum (1979) their reservations about the value of GAS, on its own, as a system for the evaluation of intervention. They both point out that GAS has not been used in strict accordance with the original specifications, and that without additional standard assessments, aggregation of client related GAS data for comparative purposes, is impossible.

The system involves the setting, by an independent team, of goals for individual clients, and specifying a range of possible outcomes, usually on a five point scale, from the worst to the best. Outcomes are specified in observable terms. At follow-up the same team, preferably, reassesses the client, using the same set of observable goals. If the rater wishes he can assign weights to each of the goals, so that those considered to be of most importance can be weighted most heavily.

A careful reading of Kiresuk & Sherman's original paper shows that, apart from the aggregation problem referred to above, they anticipated most of the likely difficulties facing the GAS user. They anticipated problems in the clear definition of goals and problems; bias in the selection of goals if clinicians were allowed to set them; the necessity to randomly assign clients to treatment groups, or to show that treatment groups do not differ at the outset.

Calsyn & Davidson report low agreement between therapists and goal-setters on client problem categories (Grygelko, Garwick & Lampan, 1973), and moderate reliability across raters of GAS scales, with correlations ranging from .85 to .51 (Baxter, 1973).

GAS scores have not been highly correlated with treatment outcomes measured by standardised instruments (Garwick, 1974). Mauger (1974), for instance, found only a .30 correlation with MMPI change scores.

Calsyn et al (1977) and Cytrynbaum (1979) found that very few (less than one fifth) of investigators using GAS, employed random assignment of clients. It was impossible to demonstrate change on the original system, and some investigators introduced baseline performance measures in the goal domains. The only way to ensure that the variation in goal-setters judgements does not introduce error into the procedure is to employ the same goal setter on each occasion and in relation to each treatment, or group, under consideration. Austin et al (1976) compared two day hospitals, one with a behavioural approach and the other a therapeutic community approach, in terms of client achievement of GAS goals after 3, 6, and 24 months. The 56 subjects were randomly selected from (but not assigned to) the two hospitals. Patients achieved more of their goals in the hospital using the behavioural approach.

Since success is assessed in terms of goals achieved, two programmes can produce the same overall performance in terms of GAS scores, but have accomplished very different objectives. Knowing that a certain proportion of the goals set in a service were achieved, is a meaningless statistic if there is no quality control on the setting of goal standards, or the measuring of change. Calsyn & Davidson propose that GAS should be used in conjunction with standard measures, so that a valid and reliable assessment is achieved. This sound proposition, likely to satisfy providers as well as funders and evaluators, has rarely been attempted.

Two benefits of GAS should be mentioned. It does encourage providers to set goals in observable terms, and it appears to generate a therapeutic effect. Cytrynbaum recommends it on the latter grounds. Calsyn et al (1977) found that 67% of GAS users in their study, used it for therapeutic purposes. Luenberger (1972) and Urban & Ford (1971), among others, have suggested that goal setting has a therapeutic value. Three controlled studies (Jones & Garwick, 1973; LaFerriere & Calsyn, 1978; and Smith, 1976) have shown that clients who are set goals using GAS have a better outcome than clients who receive therapy without goal setting.

The effectiveness of residential services in the community

It is not common to find well designed and controlled evaluations of residential services for mentally ill people. It is more common to find a wealth of material on social policy in this area backed by little or no empirical evidence (e.g Olsen, 1984). This is surprising, not least because of the growth of this sector of care, particularly private care, over the past decade. Shadish & Bootzin (1984a) suggest that the institutional setting with the most resident psychiatric patients, in the USA, is now the nursing home, not the mental hospital. Cicchinelli et al, (1981) (also in the USA) estimated that unduplicated counts of chronic patients revealed 150,000 in inpatient facilities, 350,000 with non-senile mental disorders in nursing homes, and 400,000 in nursing homes for senility without psychosis.

The House of Commons Social Services Select Committee, the Personal Social Services Research Unit, and Kathleen Jones, (in the UK) have all drawn attention to the growing problem of the growth of institutional care, and to the increasing proportion of elderly confused people in residential care, many of whom

134

might be effectively helped in their own homes. Some writers have drawn attention to the similarities between the institutional character of nursing homes and mental hospitals (Carling, 1981; Shadish & Bootzin, 1984a).

Shadish & Bootzin (1984a), on the basis of a random sample of 155 facilities, (including both hospitals and nursing homes), but with a low average return rate, concluded that they were unable to discriminate nursing homes from hospitals 'on the variables that define a total institution'. These variables were, the percentage of patients for whom the facility provided breakfast, lunch, dinner, a place to sleep, a paying job, (including sheltered work), and the percentage of time the residents spent away from the facility each day.

The number of well designed and controlled studies of outcome of residential services is very limited. It could be argued that since the objective of some services is to maintain clients in the community that 'outcome' as such, would have limited variance. This need not be the case if measures other than rehospitalisation are used, such as improvements in social functioning or role performance. It is also the case that the maintenance of a satisfied client in the community can be a good outcome, and substantial gains in performance, instrumental or social, need not always be the only objective.

An early attempt to evaluate the 'adjustment' of psychiatric patients to a residential setting in the community is Stotsky's (1967) study of discharged mental hospital patients. Stotsky investigated nursing home staff, records, and patients in two samples, one retrospective and one prospective. The retrospective sample consisted of 22 patients (from a total of 141 discharges during the year) readmitted to hospital, and 22 not readmitted. The prospective sample consisted of 65, out of a total of 68 patients consecutively placed in 28 nursing homes during a four month study period. They were followed up at 30 days and six months.

The main difference in both samples was the greater psychiatric disturbance of the rehospitalized patients. None of the variables which distinguished the nursing homes was associated with rehospitalization. 81% of those placed in the nursing home, in the prospective sample, were still there after six months. Patients whose initial reaction to the home was good, were settled in by the 30 day follow-up and remained well adjusted at six months. Only eight per cent returned to hospital, 11% died. The average age of the patients was 73, and one had been in hospital for 55 years.

Pryce (1977) took the opportunity presented by the re-wiring of a hospital ward to study the effect on the patients, of the transfer to a residential home. The broad hypothesis in this 'natural experiment' was that the transfer would lead to an increase in social stimulation, which would cause an improvement in the patient's clinical state. 40 patients were involved, 60% of whom were over 60, and they were all schizophrenia sufferers. Incontinent and physically violent patients were excluded, and the patients were randomly selected from five of the six non-geriatric wards in the hospital. About nine months later a further 27 patients with similar characteristics were selected, but these patients remained in hospital. The average age of the transferred patients was 50, and the average length of illness was 20 years, over threequarters of which had been in hospital. There were no statistically significant differences between the patients who remained in hospital and those transferred.

The results for men and women were different. Pryce summarises these as: transferred women improved clinically over two years, due to more optimistic nurse attitudes, increased work opportunities and outside contact, and reduced institutional restrictiveness; transferred men showed less clinical improvement than the women, due to some increase in outside contacts, and a marked decrease in institutional restrictiveness; women in hospital showed no clinical or social changes (except for a small decrease in ward restrictiveness); men in hospital showed some clinical improvement between 6 months and 2 years, due to increased work opportunities. The patients in the home, and those remaining in the hospital did not change their attitude to discharge; about 27% of both groups wanted to be discharged, and this % remained constant from inception to follow-up. At 6 months and 2 years, 8% and 12% of the patients in the home, wished to be transferred back to the hospital. The increased social withdrawal of the men in the home, at 6 months, is thought to be due to an overstimulating social environment. Since women were not affected in the same way, Pryce suggests that the more handicapped patients are more vulnerable to this sort of stress. He shows that on a small number of measures the men appeared to be more severely ill, and somewhat more socially handicapped.

In a review of residential care Carpenter (1978) was only able to locate two truly evaluative studies (Lamb & Goertzel, 1972; Weinman et al, 1970). The others were descriptive, or compared acute patients admitted to hospital with those diverted to community alternatives. As in Stotsky's study, most reports of residential services are focused on the patient with long-term needs.

Early studies in this area, tend to be of 'halfway houses', or similar facilities, which aimed to improve patient functioning, and were targeted at patients who could be expected to make progress in social and clinical terms. Increasingly, the later studies attend to patients with more severe and long term disability. It is important to distinguish between these two types of facility, which may have very different objectives. The confusion of the objectives of rehabilitation and maintenance has bedevilled work in this field for many years. Rog & Raush (1975) pointed out that evaluation is made difficult by 'differences among halfway houses as to goals, resident selection, programs, length of stay, and criteria for leaving the house.'

Shadish & Bootzin (1984b) acquired a random sample of 28 nursing homes, from which a subsample was selected (in an unspecified way). 163 patients with previous hospitalisation, not suffering from organic disorder or substance abuse were assessed on admission and at six month intervals for a year. Three comparison groups were similarly assessed. These groups were: 19 chronic inpatients in a CMHC ward; 22 chronic CMHC day patients ; and 18 kitchen and aide staff in the nursing homes. 82% of the patients had a diagnosis of schizophrenia.

The results showed that all three groups of psychiatric patients spent less money than the staff, staff had higher status jobs, and more social contact. The nursing home patients resembled other psychiatric patients in most respects. Over the course of the year however, the nursing home patients' levels of social integration remained static; a similar finding to Stotsky. The authors argue that this could be due to the fact that the patients were already functioning at such a low level that they could not deteriorate, or that patients might be overmedicated and understimulated. They conclude that 'nursing homes probably share too many characteristics with the old 'total institutions' to be viewed as real improvements'.

It may be that residence in a small institution in the community is an appropriate form of care for some people. The overstimulation of more independent living might result in a higher relapse rate, and readmission to a larger institution. On the other hand, they might be capable of more independent living than their present residence allows. The optimum levels of stimulation, and the optimum size of accommodation, differ for different patients. It is not possible to have one residential solution which suits all needs. Unfortunately, we have insufficient information about the optimal types of accommodation for different patients to be confident about placing people in the community. Most of current practice is based on a trial and error procedure; if there is no relapse or deterioration then providers tend to assume that error has been avoided.

A study by Slavinsky & Krauss (1982) is interesting in this context. The authors randomly assigned a group of chronic patients at a CMHC, who had been referred for long-term maintenance and support, to a medication clinic staffed by doctors, and a nurse support program. The latter combined group intervention (traditional and nontraditional group therapy, support groups and informal groups) and medication maintenance. The medication maintenance condition included attendance at a medication clinic without additional psychosocial support. 25 patients were assigned to the nursing group and 22 to the clinic. There were no clinical or demographic differences between the groups on base-line measures. Half of the patients in each group had a diagnosis of schizophrenia, and all patients were maintained on medication at the time of referral. Follow-up interviews were conducted after one and two years.

The nursing support groups met once or twice a month. Each nurse also provided continuity of care for patients assigned to the group, and telephone crisis support. Group discussions focused on problems of daily living and social competence. After one year the support group patients rated themselves as improved in their role performance, whereas the clinic group rated themselves as deteriorated. The clinic group were more satisfied than the support group, with the care they had received. Neither finding was related to baseline measures.

After two years there were no significant differences in rehospitalisation rates, but the support group had been readmitted more often (63% cf. 48%). The support group patients were significantly more agitated and more depressed; the clinic group were less agitated and depressed. The clinic group used more sources of information, radio, TV, meetings, neighbours, than the support group, and continued to spend the same amount of time out of the house as at the beginning of the study. The support group patients were spending less time out of the house at the follow-up, than at the beginning. A possible explanation is that the support group had enough social contact through the treatment programme. The groups did not differ in satisfaction with their life situation.

In terms of the care they received the support group were lukewarm about it, but the clinic group became more satisfied at each follow-up interview. Hogarty & Goldberg (1973) in a series of reports on drug treatment and sociotherapy of schizophrenia sufferers, showed that sociotherapy can interfere with medication maintenance goals. In Slavinsky & Krauss's study the same effect can be seen. One wonders about the wisdom of providing group care for a mixed group of patients, half of whom are schizophrenia sufferers. The support group patients seemed to find the intervention overstimulating, and it was unpopular. The clinic group were able to avoid overstimulation and their treatment was popular. There were, however, important differences between the groups at the outset, which clearly influenced the subsequent findings. The clinic group were already at a somewhat higher occupational level and more of the support group were living with parents. The treatment programme almost certainly compounded these differences.

While it is possible that the measures of social activity and satisfaction used in this study were inadequate to reveal important group differences, the results are consistent with our current state of knowledge. Programmes aimed at maintenance can enhance individual performance, but do so through less intrusive means, particularly with long-term patients, than the groupwork procedures chosen here. A line has to be drawn between helping disabled patients to maximise their community contacts, and putting them into overstimulating environments. This is not easy since they may be unmotivated towards improving social, occupational, and role status. Shepherd & Richardson (1979) studied four local authority day centres, and found that the approach of the management was related to the quality of personal interaction in the centres. 'Patient-oriented' management attitudes were related to a more personal approach to patients problems and an emotionally warmer quality of personal interaction. These authors did not assess the impact of these factors on client outcomes.

A survey of day services in Worcester (Tombs & Bennett, 1987) found that the main complaints about the service were about the lack of activities provided and the food. Of 478 people attending (under 65 years of age): 65% are female; 47% are between 31 and 50; 31% are single; 46% married; and only 29% are suffering from schizophrenia and affective disorder. 20% of those admitted to day care in 1984 were still attending one year later.

One way of providing less intrusive social support for people suffering from long-term problems is through 'home' or 'domiciliary care'. This type of care lies at the end of the spectrum of community services. It may take the form of providing a mixture of support services to the client in their own home (or independent living) or it may include the 'fostering' or 'family care' of the client, who lives with a selected family, on a 'boarding out' basis. In one study, by Weinman et al (1970), care was provided by workers who either visited or lived with the client. In many cases the support going into the home is needed as much by the carer as it is by the client. The care worker may be able to relieve the carer's 'unremitting burden' (Anderson, 1987) by providing continuity and information.

Weinman et al (1970) used two experimental groups and two control groups to evaluate a scheme of 'enablers', people from the same community as the client. The enablers had a good deal in common with what we currently describe as 'family aides' or 'home care workers' in the UK. One group of enablers lived in with the patients and the other visited in the traditional sense. One control group, randomly selected from the same patient population received socioenvironmental treatment, and the other received traditional hospital care. More patients in the enabler group successfully completed their treatment, and fewer were readmitted in the 24 months post treatment period. They had significantly enhanced self-esteem. The enabler program and the hospital care produced greater improvements in role performance than the socioenvironmental treatment (group therapy, skill development and enhanced social contacts).

In an uncontrolled follow-up study Pierloot & Demarsin (1976) studied the progress of 78 patients who were fostered by families over a ten year period in Geel, Belgium. Foster family care has been organized in the community of Geel for 500 years! This systematic follow-up was conducted on patients from 1968, when the procedure became a regular service, to 1977. They were a selected group, who were well maintained on medication, and not showing any dangerous behaviour. They were able to dress themselves, and were integrated into some form of occupational therapy. 28 of the 78 patients were mentally handicapped.

Only 9 patients were readmitted to hospital permanently, but only 6 returned to their family of origin. 32 patients were not rehospitalized in spite of a deteriorating psychiatric condition. 71% of the group were regarded as well integrate into their foster families, even though only 7 patients were entirely symptom free, and 29 were 'seriously disturbed'. A negative attitude towards family care was shown by 5 patients, because they had less contact with their own families, they had to work harder than when they were in hospital, or they disliked the rural area. Patients who were well integrated , had social contacts other than the family members, and went out with family members.

We have been unable to find examples of controlled studies of this form of care, nor have we found any studies of the cost-effectiveness, or cost-benefit, of this form of care. As the number of schemes of alternative residential accommodation for long-term patients increases, the need to have better data about their impact, the differences between them, and their relative cost-effectiveness, becomes all the more urgent.

Outcome studies and hidden morbidity

The costs and benefits of screening for hidden morbidity were debated by Williams (1986) and Goldberg (1986). The evidence for the effectiveness of screening is limited. A study by Johnstone & Goldberg (1976) showed that if a GP was made aware of hidden illnesses that the patients were more likely to get better quickly, and had fewer symptoms twelve months later, than patients whose illnesses were not revealed to the doctor. In a study by Hoeper et al (1984) family doctors did not alter their behaviour when given information about the patient's hidden morbidity. As Goldberg says 'If screening is to be effective, it is essential that the doctors respond in some way to the distress which has been brought to their attention' (Goldberg, 1986).

The outcome of preventive effort

Most attempts at prevention by CMHCs fall into the consultation and education category, rather than the categories of prevention of relapse, or work with high risk groups.

Reviews of studies of consultation and education do reveal that they appear to have some impact (Dowell & Ciarlo, 1983; Ozarin,1975). There is plenty of evidence that consultation services were used, particularly during the period of federal funding (Vayda & Perlmutter, 1977). However, the evidence of effectiveness is almost non-existent. Ozarin (1975) cites two studies which appear to show reductions in the number of case attending hospital and emergency services, but neither of these were controlled outcome studies.

We have been unable to locate any serious attempt to demonstrate the effectiveness of consultation and education in reduction of incidence and prevalence rates, or in the enhancement of the outcome for the clients of consultees. This absence of evidence is the single major factor in the reduction and removal of consultation and education services from the CMHC mandate in the USA. Borus writes, ' The repeal of the Mental Health Systems Act ended direct federal support of CMHCs and loosened the latter's mandate to provide consultation as an "essential service." The dismantling of regional NIMH offices has halted effective federal monitoring of CMHC efforts, ending pressure on CMHCs to solicit consultations to satisfy governmental third parties. The decrease in funding for mental health services from both federal and state sources has forced most CMHCs to focus their efforts on reimbursable direct services. Indirect services, including community consultation, have been sharply curtailed, and those consultations which have persisted are increasingly limited to agencies that can pay for the service.'(Borus, 1984).

Summary and conclusions

1

CMHCs experienced difficulty in achieving their goals before the withdrawal of federal funds made their tasks more difficult (Woy, 1981). Alterations to reimbursement practices in the US change the incentive to care for people in different settings (Taube & Burns, 1988). Without financial incentives to do so, care will not be provided in the community.

2

The use of readmission rates as outcome measures is highly dubious (Turner et al, 1979). Readmissions can represent success rather than failure, the problem for which a person is readmitted may be different from the problem at key admission, and many studies assume that community tenure is synonymous with a good outcome. Once a person is admitted then the risk of readmission is high (Sheridan & Teplin, 1981), and people assessed at CMHCs are less likely to be admitted than those assessed at a hospital, because most hospitals do not have access to alternatives. In many studies hospitalisation is treated as a homogeneous entity. Periods of 'wellness' in hospital are not reported, nor are renewed episodes of ill-health (which would be regarded as a relapse if they occurred in the community).

3

Successful services work out the proper place for hospital treatment in the spectrum of services (Tantam, 1985).

4

Adequate aftercare is essential to a successful service, but most standard aftercare provides very little contact (Solomon et al, 1983; Kirk, 1976; Goering et al, 1984). Almost half of discharged patients receive no aftercare at all, and those who do receive it infrequently.

5

Most relatives of patients experience some 'burden' but some do not report subjective burden in the presence of objective problems (Gillis & Keet, 1965; Hoenig & Hamilton, 1969). Support and information given to relatives has a powerful effect on their satisfaction with services, and their ability to cope (Hoult, 1986).

6

Goal Attainment Scaling may be a useful therapeutic technique, which enhances clinical improvement (Cytrynbaum, 1979). It is unsuitable as an evaluation technique on its own, and should be used in conjunction with other standard measures to permit comparison between subjects and aggregation of data (Calsyn & Davidson, 1978).

7

There are hardly any well designed and controlled studies of the effectiveness of residential services. Nursing homes in the community appear to have the characteristics of total institutions

(Bootzin, 1984). Some studies show increased relapse rates among patients who are put into overstimulating environments (Pryce, 1977; Slavinsky & Krauss, 1982). Home care workers appear to have considerable potential (Weinman et al, 1970).

8
There is limited evidence that screening for disorder in general practice has a beneficial effect on outcome (Johnstone & Goldberg, 1976)

9
There have been no serious attempts to demonstrate the effectiveness of primary preventive effort, even with high risk groups.

References

Anderson, R. (1987) The unremitting burden on carers. *BMJ* 94(6564):73.

Anthony, W.A. et al (1972) Efficiency of Psychiatric rehabilitation. *Psychological Bulletin*, 78:447-456.

Austin, N.K., Liberman, R.P., King, L.W. & Derisi, W.J.A. (1976) comparative evaluation of two day hospitals. *J.Nerv.Ment.Dis.* 63:253-262.

Bachrach, L. (1976) A Note on Some Recent Studies of Released Mental Hospital Patients in the Community. *Am.J.Psychiat.* 33(1):73-75.

Bachrach, L. (1977) *Deinstitutionalisation: An Analytical Review and Sociological Perspective.* Rockville, Md.NIMH.

Bachrach L (1980) Overview: Model Programs for chronic mental patients. *Am.J.Psychiat.* 137(9):1023-1031.

Barrowclough, C. & Tarrier, N. (1984) 'Psychosocial' interven tions with families and their effects on the course of schizophrenia: a review. *Psychological Medicine* 14:629-642.

Baxter, J. (1973) Combination Validity/Reliability study. *Program Evaluation Project Report*, Minneapolis.

Bayley, M. (1973) *Mental Handicap And Community Care.* RKP, London.

Bleuler, M. (1968) A 23-year longitudinal study of 208 schizophrenics and impressions in regard to the nature of schizophrenia. In D. Rosenthal & S.S.Kety *The transmission of schizophrenia* Pergamon, Oxford.

Borus, J.F. (1984) Strangers Bearing Gifts: A Retrospective Look at the Early Years of Community Mental Health Center Consultation. *Am.J.Psychiat.* 141(7):868-871.

Braun, P., Kochansky, G., Shapiro, R., Greenberg, S., Gudeman, J.E., Johnson, S. & Shore, M.F. (1981) Overview: Deinstitutionalisation of Psychiatric Patients, a Critical Review of Outcome Studies. *Am.J. Psychiat.* 138(6):736-737.

Brown, G.W.(1959) Experiences of Discharged chronic Schizophrenic Mental Hospital Patients in Various Types of Living Group. *Milbank Memorial Fund Quarterly* 37:101-131.

Brown, G.W. (1973) The mental hospital as an institution. *Soc. Sci. Med.* 7:407-424.

Brown, G.W., Birley, J.L.T. & Wing, J.K. (1972) Influence of family life on the course of schizophrenic disorders: A replication. *Brit.J.Psychiat.* 121:241-258.

Brown, G.W. & Harris, T. (1978) *The social origins of depression.* Tavistock, London.

Burvill, P. & Mittleman, M. (1971) A follow-up study of chronic Mental hospital patients. *Social Psychiatry* 6:157-171.

Calsyn, R.J. & Davidson, W.S. (1978) Do we really want a Program Evaluation Strategy Based Solely on Individualised Goals? A Critique of Goal Attainment Scaling. *Community*

Mental Health Journal 14(4):300-308.

Calsyn, R., Tornatzky, L. & Dittmar, S. (1977) Incomplete adoption of an innovation : The case of Goal Attainment Scaling. *Evaluation* 4:127-130.

Carling, P.J. (1981) Nursing Homes and chronic mental patients: a second opinion. *Schizo. Bull.* 7:574-579.

Carpenter, M.D. (1978) Residential placement for the chronic psychiatric patient: a review and evaluation of the literature. *Schizophrenia Bulletin* 4(3):384-398.

CENSIS (Centro Studi Investimenti Sociali) (1984) Le Politiche Psichiatriche Regionale nel Doporeformia e lo Stato Attuale dei Servizi. *CENSIS*, Rome.

Challis, D. & Davies, B. (1986) *Case Management in Community Care.* Gower, Aldershot.

Cicchinelli, L.F., Bell, J.C., Dittmar, N.D., Manzanares, D.L., Sackett, K.L. & Smith, G. (1981) *Factors influencing the Deinstitutionalisation of the Mentally Ill: A Review and Analysis.* Denver Research Institute, University of Denver, Denver.

Ciompi, L. & Muller, C. (1976) *Lebensweq und Alter der Schizophrenen. Eine katamnestiche Lonzeitstudies bis ins Senium.* Springer Verlag, Berlin.

Creer, C. & Wing, J.K.(1974) *Schizophrenia at home.* National Schizophrenia Fellowship, Surbiton.

Cytrynbaum, S. (1979) Goal Attainment Scaling - A critical review. *Evaluation Quarterly* 3(1):5-40.

Deane, W.N. & Brooks, G.W. (1967) Five year follow-up of chronic hospitalised patients. Vermont State Hospital, Waterbury.

Dick, P., Cameron, L., Cohen, D., Barlow, M. & Ince A. (1985) Day and Full Time Psychiatric Treatment: A controlled comparison. *Brit.J.Psychiat.* 147:246-250.

Dowell, D.A. & Ciarlo, J.A. (1983) Overview of the Community Mental Health Centres Program from an Evaluation Perspective. *Community Mental Health Journal* 19(2):95-125.

Dyck,G. (1974) The effect of a community mental health center upon state hospitalization. *Am. J. Psychiat.* 131:435-456.

Fairweather, G.W., Sanders, D.H., Cressler, D.L. & Maynard,H. (1969) *Community Life for the Mentally Ill.* Aldine, Chicago.

Falloon, I.R.H. (1985) *Family management of Schizophrenia: A Study of Clinical, Social and Family and Economic Benefits.* John Hopkins University Press, Baltimore.

Falloon, I.R.H. & Pederson, J. (1985) Family Management and the Prevention of Morbidity of schizophrenia: The adjustment of the family unit. *Brit.J.Psychiat.* 147:156-163.

Falloon, I. & Talbot, R.E. (1982) Achieving the goals of day treatment. *J.Nerv. Ment.Dis.* 170:279-284.

Fontana, A. & Dowds, B. (1975) Assessing Treatment Outcome: II the prediction of rehospitalization. J. Nerv. Ment. Dis. 161 (4):231-238.

Franklin, J.L. et al (1975) A survey of factors related to mental hospital readmissions. *Hosp. & Community Psychiat.* 11(26):749-751.

Freeman, H. & Simmons, O. (1963) *The Mental Patient Comes Home.* John Wiley & Sons, New York.

Garwick, G.(1974) A construct validity overview of Goal Attainment Scaling. *Program Evaluation Project Report,* Minneapolis.

Gillis, L.S. & Keet, M. (1965) Factors underlying the retention in the community of chronic unhospitalized schizophrenics. *B.J.Psychiat.* 111:1057-1067.

Gloag, D. (1985) Community care: rhetoric and action. *Brit. Med. Journal* 291:1372.

Goering, P., Wasylenki, D., Lancee, W. & Freeman, S.J. (1984) From Hospital to Community: Six-month and Two-year Outcomes for 505 patients. *J. Nerv. Ment. Dis.* 172(11):667-673.

Goldberg, D.P. (1986) Screening. Discussion in Shepherd M. et al (Eds) *Mental Illness in Primary Care Settings.* Tavistock, London.

Grad, J. & Sainsbury, P. (1963) Mental Illness and the Family. *Lancet* i:544-547.

Greengross, S. (1982) 'Caring for the Carers', in Glendenning, F. (ed) *Care in the Community*: Recent Research and Current Projects. University of Keele/Beth Johnson Foundation, Stoke.

Greenley, J.R. (1979) Family symptom tolerance and rehospitalization experiences of psychiatric patients. *Research in Community and Mental Health* 1:357-386.

Grygelko, M., Garwick, G. & Lampan, S. (1973) Findings of content analysis. *Program Evaluation Project Newsletter* 4:1-3.

Hammaker, R. (1983) A Client Outcome Evaluation of the Statewide Implementation of Community Support Services. *Psychosocial Rehab Journal* VII(1):2-10.

Harding, C.M., Zubin, J. & Strauss, J.S. (1987a) Chronicity in Schizophrenia: Fact, Partial Fact, or Artifact? *Hosp. & Comm. Psychiat.* 38(5):477-486.

Harding, C.M., Brooks, G.W., Ashikaga, T., Strauss, J.S. & Brier, A. (1987b) The Vermont Longitudinal Study of Persons With Severe Mental Illness: Long-Term Outcome of Subjects Who Retrospectively Met DSM-III Criteria for Schizophrenia. *Am. J. Psychiat.* 144(6):727-735.

Hatfield, A.B. (1978) Psychological costs of schizophrenia to the family. *Social Work* 355-359.

Herz,M.I., Endicott, J. & Spitzer, R.L. (1975) Brief Hospitalization of Patients with Families: Initial Results. *Am. J.Psychiat.* 132(4):413-418.

Hoenig, J. & Hamilton, M.W. (1969) *The desegregation of the mentally ill*. RKP, London.

Hoeper, E.W., Nycz, G.R., Kessler, L.G., Burke, J.D. & Pierce, W.E. (1984) The usefulness of screening for mental health. *Lancet* i:33-35.

Hogarty, G.E. & Goldberg, S.L. (1973) Drug and sociotherapy in the aftercare of schizophrenic patients: Part I. One year relapse rates. *Arch. Gen. Psychiat.* 28:54-64.

Hoult, J.(1986) Community Care of the Acutely Mentally Ill.*B. J. Psychiat.* 149:137-144.

Hoult, J. & Reynolds, I (1984) Schizophrenia: A Comparative trial of community orientated and hospital orientated psychiatric care. *Acta Psychiatrica Scandinavica* 69:359-373.

Huber, G., Gross, G. & Schuttler, R. (1979) Verlaufs und sozialpsychiatrische Langzeituntersuchungen an den 1945 bis 1959 in Bonn hospitalisierten schizophrenen Kranken. *Monographien aus dem Gesantgebiete der Psychiatrie.* Bd 21. Springer Verlag, Berlin.

Hughes, B.J. (1978) Social and clinical factors associated with burden in the families of schizophrenic patients. *M.Sc. Thesis*, University of Manchester.

Huxley, P.J. (1986) *Quality Measurement in Mental Health Services: A Discussion Paper* . GPMH, London.

Huxley, P.J. (1990) Social Work. In Freeman H. & Bennett D. (eds) *Community Psychiatry*. Churchill Livingstone, London.

Huxley, P.J., Goldberg, D.P., Maguire, G.P. & Kincey, V.A. (1979) The prediction of the course of minor psychiatric disorders. *B.J.Psychiat.* 135:535-543.

Johnstone, A. & Goldberg, D.P. (1976) Screening for psychiatric disorder in general practice. *Lancet* i:605-608.

Jones, S. & Garwick,G. (1973) Guide to goals study: goal attainment scaling as a therapy adjunct? *Program Evaluation Project Newsletter* 4(6):1-3.

Kinard, E.M. (1981) Discharged Patients Who Desire to Return to the Hospital. *Hospital & Community Psychiat.* 32(3):194-197.

Kiresuk, T.J. & Sherman, R.E. (1968) Goal Attainment Scaling: A General Method for Evaluating Comprehensive Community Mental Health Programs. *Community Mental Health Journal* 4(6):443-453.

Kiresuk, T.J. & Lund, S.H. (1975) Process and outcome measurement using Goal Attainment Scaling. In J.Zusman & C.R.Wurster (eds) *Program Evaluation: Alcohol, Drug Abuse, and Mental Health Services.* D.C. Heath & Co. Lexington, Mass.

Kirk, S.A. (1976) Effectiveness of community services for discharged mental hospital patients. *Amer.J.Orthopsychiat.* 46(4):646-659.

LaFerriere L. & Calsyn, R. (1978) Goal Attainment Scaling: An effective treatment technique in short-term therapy. *Am.J.*

Community Psychology 6:271-282.

Lamb, H.R. & Goertzel, V. (1972) High expectations of long-term ex-State hospital patients. *Am.J.Psychiat.* 129:471-475.

Lamb, H.R. & Oliphant, (1978) Schizophrenia through the eyes of families. *Hospital & Community Psychiatry* 29:803-806.

Langsley, D., Machotka, P. & Flomenhaft, K. (1971) Avoiding mental hospital admission: a follow-up study. *Am.J.Psychiat.* 127:1391-1394.

Lavender, A. (1987) Improving the Quality of Care on Psychiatric rehabilitation wards. *B.J.Psychiat.* 150:476-481.

Luenberger, M.C. (1972) Therapeutic Movement as a function of awareness of goals. *Unpublished Doctoral Dissertation*, University of California.

Mann, A.H. Jenkins, R. & Belsey, E. (1981) The twelve month outcome of patients with neurotic illness in general practice. *Psychological Medicine* 11:535-550.

Mauger, P.(1974) A study on the construct validity of goal attainment scaling. *Program Evaluation Project Report*, Minneapolis.

Moroney, R.M. (1976) *The Family & The State*. Longman,London.

Mosher,L.R., Menn, A. & Matthews, S. (1975) evaluation of home based treatment for schizophrenia. *Am.J. Orthopsychiat.* 45:455-467.

Ochberg, F.M. (1976) Community Mental Health Center Legislation: Flight of the Phoenix. *Am.J.Psychiat.* 133(1):56-61.

Olsen, R. (1984) (ed) *Social Work And Mental Health*. Tavistock, London.

Ozarin, L. (1975) Community Mental Health: Does it work? Review of the Evaluation Literature. In W.T. Barton & C.J.Sandborn (eds) *An Assessment of the Community Mental Health Movement*. D.C. Heath, Lexington, Mass.

Ozarin, L. (1978) The pros and cons of case-management. In J.A.Talbott (ed) *The Chronic Mental Patient*. American Psychiatric Association, Washington.

Pasamanick, B., Scarpitti, F.R., Lefton, M., Dinitz, S., Werner, J.J. & McPheeters, H. (1964) Home vs Hospital care for Schizophrenics. *J. Am. Med. Assoc.* 187:177-181.

Paul, G.L. & Lentz, R. (1977) *Psychosocial Treatment of Chronic Mental Patients*. Camb. Mass. Harvard University Press.

Pierloot,R.A. & Demarsin, M. (1976) Family care versus hospital stay for chronic psychiatric patients. *H.C.Psych.*217-224.

Pryce, I.G.(1977) The effects of social changes in chronic schizophrenia: a study of forty patients transferred from hospital to residential home. *Psych. Med.* 7:127-139.

Reynolds, I. & Hoult, J.E. (1984) The relatives of the mentally ill. A comparative trial of community-oriented and hospital-oriented psychiatric care. *J.Nerv.Ment.Dis.* 172(1): 480-489.

Riessman, E., Rabkin, J.G. & Struening, E.L. (1977) Brief versus standard psychiatric hospitalization: A critical review of the literature. *Community Mental Health Review* 2:1-10.

Rog, D.J. & Raush, H.L. (1975) The psychiatric halfway house: How is it measuring up? *Community Mental Health Journal* 11:155-162.

Rosenblatt, A. & Mayer, J. (1974) Recidivism of mental patients: a review of past studies. *Amer.J. Orthopsychiat.* 44(5):697-706.

Rutlege, L. & Binner, P. (1970) Readmissions to a Community Mental Health Center. *Community Mental Health Journal* 6(2):136-143.

Sartorious, N., Jablensky, A. & Shapiro, R. (1977) Two year follow-up of the patients in the WHO International Pilot Study of Schizophrenia. *Psychological Medicine* 7:529-541.

Shadish, W.R. & Bootzin, R.R. (1984a) Nursing Homes: The New Total Institution in Mental Health Policy. *Int.J.Partial Hospitalization* 2(4):251-262.

Shadish, W.R. & Bootzin, R.R. (1984b) The social integration of Psychiatric patients in nursing homes. *Am.J. Psychiat.* 141(10):1203-1207.

Shepherd, G. & Richardson, A. (1979) Organisation and interaction in psychiatric day centres. *Psych. Med.* 9:573-579.

Sheridan, E. & Teplin, L. (1981) Recidivism in Difficult Patients: Differences Between Community Mental Health Center and State Hospital Admissions. *Am.J.Psychiat.* 138(5):688-690.

Slavinsky, A.T. & Krauss, J.B. (1982) Two approaches to the management of long-term psychiatric outpatients in the community. *Nursing Research* 31(5):284-289.

Smith, D.L. (1976) Goal Attainment Scaling as an adjunct to counselling. *J.of Counselling Psychology* 23:22-27.

Solomon, P., Gordon, B. & Davis, J.M. (1983) An Assessment of Aftercare Services Within a Community Mental Health System. *Psychosocial Rehabilitation Journal* 7(2):33-39.

Solomon, P., Gordon, B. & Davis, J. (1984) Differentiating Psychiatric Readmissions from Nonreadmissions. *Amer. J. Orthopsychiat.* 54(3):426-435.

Stein, L. & Test, M.A. (1980) Alternative to Mental Hospital treatment I:Conceptual model, treatment programme and clinical evaluation. *Archives of General Psychiatry* 37:392-397.

Stotsky, B.A (1967) A controlled study of factors in the successful adjustment of mental patients to nursing homes. *Am.J.Psychiat.* 123(10):1243-1251.

Strauss, J.S. & Carpenter, W.T. (1974) The prediction of outcome in schizophrenia II. Relationships between predictor and outcome variables. *Arch. Gen. Psychiat.* 32(1):37.

Stubblebine, J.M. & Decker, J.B. (1971) Are Urban Mental Health Centers Worth It? Part II. *Am.J.Psychiat.* 128:480-483.

Tansella, M., De Salvia, D. & Williams, P. (1987) The Italian psychiatric reform: some quantitative evidence. *Social Psychiatry* 22:37-48.

Tansella, M. & Williams, P. (1987) Editorial: The Italian experience. *Psychological Medicine* 17:283-289.

Tantam (1985) Alternatives to Psychiatric Hospitalization. *B.J.Psychiat.* 146:1-4.

Test, M.A. (1981) Effective Community Treatment of the Chronically Mentally Ill: What is Necessary? *Journal of Social Issues* 37(3):71-86.

Test, M.A. & Stein, L.I.(1980) Alternative to mental hospital treatment. III Social Cost. *Arch. Gen. Psychiat.* 37:409-412.

Thompson, J.W. et al (1982) Past- now 50 years of psychiatric services 1940-1990. *Hosp. & Comm. Psychiat.* 33:711-717.

Tombs, D. & Bennett, C. (1987) The Evaluation of the Worcester Development Project. *Int.J.Soc.Psychiat.* 33(2):92-98.

Tsuang, M.T., Woolsen, R.F. & Fleming, J.A. (1979) Long term outcome of major psychoses, I: schizophrenia and affective disorders compared with psychaiatrically symptom free surgical conditions. *Arch Gen. Psychiat.* 36:1295-1301.

Turner,A.J. (1979) Readmission rates to Community Mental Health Centers as a measure of programme effectiveness. *Evaluation and the Health Professions* 1(5):20-31.

Tyrer, P., Remington, M. & Alexander, J. (1987) The outcome of neurotic disorders after outpatient and day hospital care. *B.J.Psychiat.* 151:57-62.

Urban, H.B. & Ford, D.H. (1971) Some historical and conceptual perspectives on psychotherapy and behaviour change. In S.E. Bergin & S.L.Garfield (Eds) *Handbook of psychotherapy and behaviour change*. New York, John Wiley.

Vaughn, C.E. & Leff, J.P. (1976) The influence of family and social factors on the course of psychiatric illness.*Brit.J.Psychiat.* 129:125-137.

Vayda, A.M. & Perlmutter, F.D. (1977) Primary prevention in Community Mental Health Centers: A Survey of Current Activity. *Community Mental Health Journal* 13:343-351.

Weinman, B., Sanders, R., Kleiner, R. & Wilson, S. (1970) Community based treatment of the chronic psychotic. *Comm.Ment.Health Journal* 6:13-21.

Wenger, G.C. (1984) *The Supportive Network: Coping with Old Age.* Allen & Unwin, London.

Wessler, R.L. & Iven, D. (1970) Social Characteristics of Patients Readmitted to a Community Mental Health Center. *Comm. Mental Health Journal* 6(1):69-74.

Wilkinson, G. (1984) Day care for patients with psychiatric disorders. *B.M.J.* 288:1710-1712.

Wilkinson, G. (1985) Community care: planning mental health services. *B. M. J.* 290:1371-1373.

Wing,J.K., Carstairs, G.M., Monck, E. & Brown, G.W. (1964) Morbidity in the community of schizophrenic patients discharged from London Mental Hospitals in 1959. *Brit. J.Psychiat.* 110:10.

Wittenborn, J.R., McDonald, D.C. & Maurer, H.S. (1977) Persisting symptoms in schizophrenia predicted by background factors. *Arch. Gen. Psychiat.* 34:1057-1061.

Woy, J.R., Wasserman, D.B. & Weiner-Pomerantz, R. (1981) Community Mental Health Centres: Movement away from the model. *Community Mental Health Journal* 17:265-276.

6 Accountable services

Introduction

Before embarking on a discussion of accountability, it is worth reviewing the major goals of the CMHC programme in the USA. Dowell and Ciarlo (1983) have identified nine goals:-

To increase the range and quantity of public mental health services (pertinent issues include volume of services, increased number of specialised services; maintenance of a community mental health orientation, and fiscal viability of the centres)
To make services equally available and accessible to all (issues involve income groups, minority-majority, young-old, and urban-rural dimensions).
To provide services in relation to the existing needs in the community (includes issues about services to high-need populations and severely disabled patients).
To decrease state hospital admissions and residents (issues concern reduced admissions due to CMHC's and appropriateness of community replacements).
To maximise citizen participation in community programmes.
To prevent development of mental disorders (includes evidence for effectiveness of prevention and weakness of preventive efforts in practice).
To coordinate mental health services in the catchment area (includes continuity of care and services to other agencies).
To provide services as efficiently as possible (includes cost of

mental health services in CMHC's and efficiency problems).
To provide services that reduce suffering and increase personal functioning (issues include the evidence for effectiveness of community mental health services, and the development of methods for improving services).

Dowell & Ciarlo concluded that the most significant achievement of the CMHC programme in the USA was the increase in the quantity and range of public mental health services. Equality of access to services was also improved but all inequities were not removed. Problems continue to exist in funding services on the basis of need, in providing services to what they call 'chronic clients', and in co-ordinating services. Prevention efforts suffered from uncertainties and perhaps overly optimistic expectations.

Accountability and community mental health

Accountability for a mental health worker's activity is often related to more than one source. It may be to a combination of 'stakeholders' who have different interests and different degrees of power over the actions of the worker. The main stakeholders involved in the delivery of mental health services appear to be:-

The employees' managing agency
The professional body (or bodies) of which the employee is a member
The workers who share responsibility with an individual employee for the delivery of services
The people using services and their carers (usually families)
The communities (or their representatives) within which services are delivered.

In this review we will concentrate on the last two lines of accountability. The literature reflects the fact that these are now considered to be the areas in most need of attention. The first three stakeholders will be dealt with briefly.

The employee's managing agency

Traditionally accountability to the employing agency has been the most powerful influence on the worker, whether nurse, social worker, psychologist, etc. It is the employing agency that pays the wage and that has the power to suspend or dismiss the worker in the event of unsatisfactory conduct. Mental health workers in the community are held accountable in the same way as they were when they were based in hospital, but the mechanisms for ensuring accountability are different. Accountability in the community is frequently assessed a s part of a process called 'evaluation.' Lebow (1982) identifies five models for evaluating services at community mental health centres:

(a) The organisational model

This model focuses on the management of the facility. Its roots are in industrial engineering, its proponents are largely management personnel and its zeitgeist resembles that of most businesses. This model assumes the appropriateness and viability of the organisational structure, the scope of the operation, the efficiency of management, the quality of services provided, and the relation of the services to community need and demand.

The assessment of organisational functioning includes several domains. One is the assessment of structure. Elements that may be assessed include institutional accreditation, type of programmes available, amount of money spent, adequacy of the organisational table, quality of practitioners training, quality assurance efforts, and opportunities for staff development. In addition to structural assessment, the organisational model applies utilization and continuity measures. Utilization measures determine the quantity of services offered and the productivity of staff, programmes, and facilities. Utilization data may also be combined with community need or demand data to determine availability of service (number of services in relation to population) and accessibility of service for various groups of community residents. Continuity measures determine the movement patterns of clients within the care system.

Unfortunately organisational data do not provide a complete description of the quality, effectiveness and comparability of services. There are specific problems with each form of organisational data. Utilization data may be reported in different units, which make comparability a problem. Structural assessment must depend on generally stated standards that may or may not be relevant in specific instances. Further, structural criteria necessarily accentuate the more easily measurable aspects of a facility, and thus may emphasise insignificant aspects of the service.

(b) The care process model

In this model, the quality of services is compared with some standard of practice. This model focuses on appropriate consignment of clients to services and the effectiveness of service delivery. Its principal strength lies in its assessments of the actual behaviour of practitioners.

Several problems plague the model. Clinicians are reluctant to open treatment to examination; there are constraints of confidentiality and cost. CMHC records rarely represent an accurate,

154

or easily accessible source of data.

(c) The consumer-evaluation model

This model derives from marketing research and focuses on the consumer's opinions about services offered. These consumers may either be clients who assess services they have received or residents of the community who assess the service system as a whole; most research has investigated client satisfaction.

Community acceptability of services is an important factor in determining the utilization and funding of services; the satisfaction of clients is an important determinant of utilization, a mediating goal in the pursuit of treatment effectiveness, and an ultimate goal of treatment in its own right. Consumer-evaluation methods are direct and inexpensive.

Distortion in reports is a major problem. The consumer's assessment may be altered by a desire to maintain social desirability, by acquiescence to the positive phrasing of questions, by cognitive dissonance, by the filtering of specifics through a positive halo response, or by reactivity (alteration of behaviour due to awareness of being evaluated). Such assessment is not a direct measure of service quality. Clients may be affected by positive or negative transference, poor reality testing, and a lack of knowledge about the elements that constitute appropriate treatment.

(d) The efficacy model

This model evaluates the clinicians' performance in changing clients and consultees. The model has its roots in clinical trials research. Measures of change may assess psychiatric symptomatology, general role functioning, or may focus on the specific goals of treatment, e.g. target complaints. Information may be gathered from various sources: the client, the therapist, significant others, independent raters.

The model's basic strength is that of testing the stated purpose of most services -the facilitation of change in clients and consultees. The principal problems are the pragmatic difficulties of measuring outcome and the precarious nature of the relationship between treatment and outcome. Change is difficult to measure and measures from alternative perspectives often intercorrelate poorly. Efficacy measures remain subject to many problems in validation e.g. the influence of reactivity, cognitive dissonance, and desire for social acceptance must be assessed. Considerable progress has been made over the past decade in the standardisation of efficacy assessments and relevant and appropriate statistical techniques are increasingly available.

(e) The community-impact model

This model assesses the CMHC's influence on the community as a whole. Measures of impact include the community's knowledge of services. The model's difficulties are an extension of those with outcome. Community mental health is even harder to measure than that of individual clients, and is seldom employed as a measure of centre functioning. Straightforward measures of community impact (e.g. knowledge of the centre) can be of value for certain purposes.

To summarise, the organisational model focuses on organisation functioning and the ability to offer service, the care-process model on the care delivered, the consumer-evaluation model on the acceptability of care, the efficacy model on the outcome of care, and the impact model on the effects on the community.

Ciarlo (1982) suggests that 'accountability' has been increasingly differentiated in the literature in service utilization studies, attainment of process goals, cost studies, client outcome studies, and community impact studies. This author suggests that two types of programme accountability had tended to dominate CMHC programmes, the 'performance measurement' type at the federal and state level, and the 'quality assurance' type at the local level.

Under the 'performance measurement' umbrella, Ciarlo suggests that five objectives and associated indicators had been developed for use in the CMHC: financial validity, efficiency/productivity, accessibility of care, continuity of care, and quality assurance activities. Local 'quality assurance' accountability is said to be virtually synonymous with peer review. Ciarlo pointed out that the programme had been in existence for some time before there was a 'wave' of 'client outcome' studies. Such studies include analysis of psychological well being; social well being in family, job and community; and client satisfaction with treatment programmes. Ciarlo found that mental health 'officials and legislators' listed the following items of major importance for managers concerned with accountability:

Identifying criteria for measuring outcomes of mental health programmes.
Forecasting or predicting demands for services or funds.
Finding agreement between legislators and mental health executives on common definitions and terms.
Increasing information while simplifying reporting requirements.
Right to treatment versus right to refuse treatment.
Lack of clarity about the type and limits of each actor's accountability.

Ciarlo analysed the results of other studies of American policy-makers to support his thesis. A study of 336 policy makers suggested that the two accountability measures (of 15 types of mental health system accountability listed) which are most directly concerned with 'client outcome' are the 'safe and effective' and 'measurement of patient improvement' categories, should together be given the highest priority in future arrangements. This indicates a concern which moves beyond the simple demand for cost-effective services.

The professional body of which the employee is a member

This has traditionally been a fairly weak line of accountability for workers, although professional bodies have been involved with the setting of standards and the development of ethical codes. The creation of new professions and associated professional bodies (community psychiatric nurses, community psychologists, community occupational therapists) have contributed to the interdisciplinary tensions and struggles for power footholds in community mental health. These tensions have been frequently noted in the literature. A good example of the literature on issues of responsibility, authority and accountability from the viewpoint of a particular profession is a recent publication by the British Psychological Society (1986). The paper seeks to explore accountability by linking it to the notion of responsibility and clarifying the different types of responsibility which exist.

The workers who share responsibility with an individual employee for the delivery of services

The 'teamwork' spirit fostered in the community mental health movement was partly driven by the requirement of a coordinated service. One implication of this newfound teamwork was the demand for workers to be accountable to one another in their teams. Teams wanted operational policies which reflected this new sense of inter-professional accountability. The concept of responsibility, especially that of medico-legal responsibility, became a focus of concern as a lack of clarity existed about the extent of medical responsibility for patient care in non-institutional settings. Øvertveit (1986) explores in depth the issues of organising workers from different backgrounds in multidisciplinary teams and the implications for accountability. These issues were also taken up by the D.H.S.S. (1980) in the 'Nodder Report', where clarification was given on the thorny issue of the 'medico-legal' responsibilities of consultant psychiatrists. The report concluded that:

> there is, as we understand it, no basis in law for the common-ly expressed idea that a consultant may be held responsible

for negligence on the part of others simply because he is the 'responsible medical officer'; or that, though personally blameless, he may be held commander. A multi-disciplinary team has no 'commander' in this sense .

The accountability of consultants is also said to be unclear and many people are dissatisfied with the present uncertainty. Among the proposals to clarify the position are, the use of short term contracts and the use of peer review.

The people using services and their carers

Along with the growth of non-institutional intervention came new demands for mental health workers to be made answerable for their actions to people on the receiving end of services. The growth of the 'consumer movement' in mental health mirrored the general impact of consumerism in the United States during the 1960's and 1970's following Nader's work on the unaccountable activity of American corporate power (Peck,1986). (For a discussion of Nader's influence on the community mental health movement, see Chu (1974)).

Health care consumption is a very different form of consumerism from that of cash exchange for an industrially-manufactured product. Payment through taxation or insurance schemes is not the same as payment over the counter; the professional knowledge base of health care workers is not as easily questioned as the craftmanship behind poorly-manufactured goods; the emotional response of a sick person to those providing care is likely to be very different from that of a customer buying an ordinary service from a tradesperson; and finally the health care process has a unique set of laws and professional and voluntary codes which affect its delivery (Taylor 1983).

Despite such differences, health service consumerism became a powerful current within the community mental health movement. The 'Short Report' (Social Services Committee 1985) gave a boost to U.K. consumerism in its list of recommendations: "We recommend that all agencies responsible ensure that plans for services are devised with, as well as for mentally disabled people and their families' (para 31); "We recommend that the Department lay an obligation on authorities to ascertain so far as practicable, and give due consideration to, the wishes and feelings of mentally disabled individuals for whom a service is provided, and in particular where closure of a long-stay facility is contemplated. We also recommend that efforts be made to facilitate the participation of individual mentally disabled in the planning and management of services" (para 149).

Consumerism, client choice and self-determination are also discussed in a Personal Social Services Research Unit publication (P.S.S.R.U. 1987) Consumer centred literature has been around

in the voluntary sector for many years (Brandon 1981). Administrators and mental health workers saw potential gains from
client involvement in the mental health system and in the creation of alternative services. One author (Kopolow 1981) specified
7 potential benefits: increased sense of client self-esteem; increased optimism about recovering; development of innovative
programmes more responsive to the needs of clients; decreased
cost; creation of a community-based force of advocates for improved mental health services; provision of services to underserved populations; improved public image.

Mental health workers found themselves confronted with
demands for participation from people using services in all aspects of service policy and service delivery. Altman (1978) identified 11 policy areas with potential for resident participation in
institutional settings. But involvement was not to be confined to
institutional settings. The involvement of user and ex-user activists took several forms, including: input to agency policy and
budget control; service provision by users themselves; systems of
advocacy, advice and representation; surveys and evaluation
studies involving people using services; education of planners and
mental health workers; protest and pressure group activity; and
litigation.

Client satisfaction surveys

During the late 1970's and 1980's a number of scales were developed which aimed to assess patients' views of services (Essex
et al 1981; Glenn 1975; Larsen et al 1979; Love et al 1979; Slater
et al 1982). These scales concentrated on satisfaction with care.
Windle and Paschall (1981) found that, of 103 client satisfaction
instruments received in 1980, only five of 103 appear to have
been developed by citizens/consumers.

Fisher (1983) has pointed out that satisfaction surveys have
some serious drawbacks. That there is a tendency for respondents to express a high degree of satisfaction with just about
everything in areas of life where satisfaction ratings are taken;
some clients do not distinguish satisfaction with the way a service is given from satisfaction with the adequacy of the service
itself; it is difficult to distinguish in reports of satisfaction exactly
who is satisfied - different family members may have different
views; and ratings of satisfaction relate primarily to the quality of
the contact between worker and client, not to its outcome.

A very different approach to satisfaction could be to concentrate on remedies for unsatisfactory care. Colom (1981) has suggested that sophisticated grievance policies should be developed
in order to correct deficiencies of user participation in evaluation.
Such procedures should be time-limited; accessible; understandable; usable; protective of the rights of clients; and informative.

In addition, policies should identify an external advocate for the client. On a more general level, this author argues that client representation can be obtained by the placement of clients as equal and valued members on federal, state and local boards. He suggests that this requires the active recruitment, orientation and training of clients in regard to the mental health and social service delivery systems to ensure informed participation as well as the training of clients for their empowerment to serve as advocates, self-advocates and members of boards whose function is the evaluation, planning and implementation of mental health programmes.

Windle and Paschall examined complaint systems. They found that between 1972 and 1979 the proportion of community mental health centres reporting use of a client complaints system rose from 10% to 48%. The authors suggest three reasons for the state of affairs where client involvement is passive rather than active. Firstly, CMHC's have concentrated on technical aspects of evaluation (refinement of instruments, etc.). The larger question of who should be involved, and how, are rarely considered. Secondly, it is difficult to engage clients actively. Many implementation issues are rarely addressed, such as how to identify consumers who are willing and able to invest time in such an endeavour, how to co-ordinate this effort with professional effort, and how to convince staff that this endeavour will have benefits for the centres. Finally, client involvement in evaluation may be seen as encroachment on professional ground.

Kaufmann et al (1979) describe the development of a client survey instrument which attempted to synthesise the interests of consumers, citizens and administrators. Over 80 client satisfaction surveys used in other programmes were reviewed and 38 sample questions extracted. Members of each group - consumers, CMHC citizen advisory board members and CMHC administrators - were asked to examine the list with an instruction to extract items where they thought it would be particularly helpful to know the opinions of clients. The groups did not agree about the kinds of questions that were desirable. The consumers showed great interest in gathering clients' opinions about confidentiality and links with other agencies, while the other groups tended to ignore these topics. The authors created a survey instrument that included high-priority items from each group. The survey was then completed by 205 out-patients.

Areas of general agreement included impact of treatment (91% felt that services had helped them), overall satisfaction (87% were satisfied), confidentiality (81% felt that it was important and 90% felt that the programme kept their problems confidential), and follow-up (86% would like their therapists to telephone them shortly after they stopped treatment). There was no clear client preference about family involvement in therapy or ethnic matching of therapist with client.

Service provision by users and ex-users

Kopolow (1981) comments: 'Members of the ex-patient movement in recent years have become increasingly vocal in demand-
ing changes in society's behaviour toward those labelled mentally
ill and especially in mental health professionals' treatment of this
population. While individual ex-patient groups differ in strategies
(some follow the complete abolition of the existing mental health
system, while others feel that major changes in staff attitudes
and more responsive services are the best approaches to follow),
they share a common opposition to forced treatment and a belief
in the value of patient input and direction of mental health services.'

Kopolow goes on to suggest that such impact has been rare in
the American CMHC movement. Among the obstacles faced by
ex-patients in trying to set up patient-run alternatives is the
serious problem of the difficulty in obtaining adequate funding.
Chamberlin (1979) has pin-pointed the sophisticated accounting
and management procedures and organisational systems generally required by funding bodies, as major hurdles for the loose
structure and innovative style of self-help programmes. His
analysis of the US scene was that only a relatively few ex-patient
programmes existed, and of these number, only a handful were
affiliated with CMHC's.

Kopolow describes three major types of ex-patient operations.
The first is independent self-help. This is defined as 'any organised group of people and programmes run by present and former
patients for the benefit and assistance of those individuals whose
behaviour, beliefs or felt problems are considered by society to
reflect mental illness.' Chamberlin (1979) explains that programmes created by the ex-patient movement offer support,
friendship, and tolerance in lieu of psychotherapy, medication or
a structural milieu. Recovery, Inc is cited by Kopolow as an
example of this type of participation. Recovery (The Association
of Nervous and Former Mental Patients) was founded in 1937
and has operated as a freestanding lay-run alternative mental-
health resource since 1952.

It has established clear motives and policy guidelines for
recruiting, training and socialising its lay self-help group leaders,
all of whom are typified as either 'nervous persons' or former
mental patients. In 1984 that there were over 1,000 Recovery
self-help groups and 7,000 dues-paying members at that date.
Members do not leave to pay dues nor have to be referred by a
professional. Of a sample of 393 Recovery leader-administrators,
group leaders and 'helpers', 72% were women, 99.7% were white,
62.5% were middle-aged (defined as 40-60 years old), and 74.5%
were married. The sample had received 'above-average' education (47% college educated), 52.5% had been previously hospitalised for mental illness, and about 90% had been treated with

drugs or medicines for a nervous problem.

Another frequently cited independent self help group is the Mental Patients' Association of Vancouver (established in 1971), described by Kopolow(1981) as an 'organisation of ex-patients which operates a 7-day a week drop-in centre and 5 co-operative residences, all on the principle of participatory democracy. All decision-making powers are in the hands of the membership and are expressed by votes taken at weekly business meetings.'

Kopolow's second category is the collaborative programme. This category refers to ex-patient groups pursuing joint projects with CMHC staff. Kopolow suggests that such ventures promote public recognition of the value of ex-patient groups and help them to attract funding. However, the ex-patient groups may find themselves diluting their aims or toning down their political activism in order to avoid losing financial support. CMHC's may have problems as well if they are seen to be funding controversial or activist programmes. An example quoted is that of the San Fernando CMHC, California, which 'makes extensive use of volunteers, including ex-patients, and has established a number of self help groups and friendship clubs.' On a visit to the USA in 1989 the author observed very successful examples of this type of venture. Ex-patients in Boulder, Colorado are employed as mental health workers and in other parts of the mental health service. A special training program for ex-patients wishing to become case managers was established by the State mental health department, and one was working successfully as a member of the community support service. Others were engaged with CMHC staff on the development of housing provision.

The third category is the advocacy programme. According to Kopolow 'all advocates should share a common loyalty to their clients and adherence to the mission of assisting the clients in obtaining all the rights and entitlements to which they have a claim .... The advocate serves as an extension of the client - a force striving to ensure that the client's perspective, priorities and needs are addressed'. Kopolow identifies four areas in which he believes ex-patient advocates have mainly directed their efforts. These are: increased public understanding of the concerns of those labelled 'mental patient'; the protection of the legal rights of clients and assurance of their entitlements under existing Federal, State and local programmes; raising clients' consciousness (eg by distributing literature, giving advice and information about aspects of the mental health system); and mutual support programmes for present and former patients.

The communities (or their representatives) within which services were delivered

US Public Law 88-164 (Mental Retardation Facilities and

CMHC's Construction Act of 1963) required that state agencies taking advantage of the legislation create state advisory councils to include 'representatives of consumers of the services provided by such facilities' but did not define consumers or specify numbers to be involved. Later legislation, Public Law 89-749, relating to comprehensive health planning (comprehensive Health Planning and Public Health Service Amendments of 1966), was more detailed in its requirements for consumer representation on the state health planning councils, stating that a 'majority of the membership of such councils shall consist of representatives of consumers of health services'. The Community Mental Health Centre Amendments Act of 1975 legislated requirements to include residents of the catchment area in the review of centers' statistics and evaluations and to include demographic representation of the catchment area in community mental health centres governing or advisory boards.

Thomson (1973) points out that the words 'consumer' and 'citizen' were frequently used interchangeably in the early literature in community participation. Two key stakeholders are, however, to be distinguished. The first is the person who is a user or ex-user of mental health services or a relative of a service user. Accountability to this group has been dealt with in the preceding section. The second is the person who has not used mental health services but is a potential user and has some interest in representing the catchment community being served by a community mental health facility. It is the latter group who were usually found as members of CMHC 'citizen boards of control'. However, the distinction is not a clear one because actual users or ex-users of mental health services were often subsumed under the category of community representatives and were to be found on CMHC citizen boards.

Roman and Schmais (1972) have characterised the community boards which developed as a consequence of US Federal legislation, promoting community participation in a range of fields during the 1960's, under five general types according to their formal role:-

(i) The Incorporated Body model: This is a legally viable structure where the objective is maximum community participation and control. In this case, the board contracts for the services of administrative and professional staff.

(ii) The Delegated Authority model: A board that encourages this model typically receives complete operating authority from a prime contractor. The latter, however, retains administrative and professional personnel on its own staff.

(iii) The Shared Responsibility model: This model is based on a commitment from administration and professionals to work with the community board. Legal responsibility is vested in the central affiliated institution.

163

(iv) The Issue Delegation model: legal responsibility again reposes in the institutional staff, but decision-making authority on specifically delegated matters is reserved for the community board. The extent of community input is considerably attenuated.

(v) The Purely Advisory model: This is the most prevalent model. Under this model the community board holds neither legal nor de facto power or control over agency policy.

Nassi (1978) outlined 3 major obstacles to community control in mental health centres: the role of professionalism, mental health ideology, which tends to be exclusive and devaluing; and the mental health power structure, the parallel bureaucratic agencies which, by virtue of their control over professional and financial resources, co-operate in their own mutual support and maintain the decision making power within the field.

Roman and Schmais (1972) characterise the cluster of problems that have typically afflicted participation-oriented facilities. These include: conflict between community and agency concerning the nature and degree of participation; manipulation of community representatives and/or employees by professional staff and administrators; ineffective community participation resulting from lack of political/bargaining skills or issue expertise; and frustration of community workers and non-professionals when no structured means of advancement is available, either within the agency or to other programmes.

The authors suggest that four factors will play a part in the development of viable programmes:-

A network of governance that ensures the accountability of administrative and professional staff to governing board; of governing board to catchment area constituency

A continuing effort to build in and sustain a 'politically resilient structure that moves towards an increasing level of stability through effective bargaining mechanisms'

A sharp but operationally feasible demarcation between policy and service components, while providing governing committees with appropriate technical assistance, to reduce the frequency of largely nonsubstantive conflicts between agency and consumers

A structured, explicit and reality-oriented career advancement programme that responds to the specific needs of poverty populations, while contributing to the overall service delivery capability of the service.

Riley (1981) suggests that community participation in service delivery can be made operational in at least three ways: the use of volunteers, the use of clients as service deliverers, and the employment of individuals identified with clients through cultural similarity and social activism on their behalf (paraprofessionals).

Volunteers can be as effective as mental health workers (Siegel 1973) but little is known of how well they perform as representatives of the community in service delivery. Paraprofessionals are frequently said to have a special sense of communality that facilitates the positive outcome of interventions in mental health settings and are often viewed as effective social activists because of their unique appreciation of local social conditions. Giving them a career structure is seen as a way to create valued work opportunities for people in poor communities.

Riley (1981), in assessing current practice, suggested that approximately 10% of staff positions in CMHC's are volunteer status and that 53% of all volunteers were paraprofessionals. Paraprofessionals are often defined by three criteria which are used interchangeably: by their education (be lack of clinical qualifications), the activities they engage in (the level and type of work performed), and their residence (population from which they are drawn). Reiff and Riessman (1965) make a distinction between ubiquitous and indigenous paraprofessionals. The former have typically similar class background as professionals, the latter a similar background as their clients. Language, values and attitudes are respectively different.

Durlak (1979) reviewed 42 studies and found that paraprofessionals achieve clinical outcomes equal to or better than that obtained by professionals. However, the criticism was made that paraprofessionals were selectively recruited, co-opted into the values of the CMHC and hence lost their special representative function. Although there is a body of literature on the effectiveness of paraprofessionals, the U.S. National Institute of Mental Health (NIMH) data omits detailed reference to their socio-cultural characteristics or work functions and so it is hard to know how much their job includes explicit representation of community values in service delivery.

Riley et al (1980) studied 20 CMHC's to determine the extent of social activist roles among CMHC workers. Two measures of activism were obtained: the workers perception of what the organisation expects (CMHC Activism) and what the worker would prefer to do if free from constraints (Preferred Activism). Neither of these two forms of activism were strongly held by paraprofessional workers as a group. Further, there were no reliable differences between paraprofessionals and any professional group on CMHC Activism. Paraprofessionals differed only from medically-trained personnel (the lowest-scoring professional group) on Preferred Activism. In other words, the evidence suggests that paraprofessionals failed to inject the note of community activism with CMHC service delivery that was expected.

Riley concludes that citizen participation in service delivery is poorly conceptualised, the greatest failure being lack of specific techniques by which it is to be achieved and cultivated. Among the alternative explanations for the finding that paraprofessionals seem limited in how much activism they bring into CMHC's are the following: the belief that indigenous paraprofessionals favour activism is misguided and requires reconsideration; the information available does not permit meaningful conclusions because several classes of workers have been lumped together.

Citizen participation in evaluation

The other major area of citizen participation in CMHC is the field of evaluation. Windle and Paschall (1981) report on the incidence of client participation in CMHC evaluation in the United States. They refer to evidence from 1979 that 81% of 287 responding CMHC's reported that they had assessed client satisfaction over the preceding 12 months, a much higher rate than in 1972. However, although the incidence of client feedback evaluation was increasing, there was poor involvement of people using services in both the development and administration of testing materials:

Table 6.1 Number of client satisfaction studies, by groups which developed and administered the measures:

		DEVELOPED BY		
		Agency alone	Agency citizen/ consumer collaboration	Citizens/ consumers alone
	Agency alone	56	2	0
ADMIN- ISTERED BY	Agency-citizen/ consumer involvement	2	0	1
	Citizen/ consumer alone	0	1	1

It is clear from the table that lay citizens and people using mental health services have little active part in either the development or administration of the rating scales. Windle (1979) has gathered empirical evidence that having the public involved in evaluation or made aware of findings done increase the likelihood that the findings will be used. Dinkel et al (1981) suggest that citizen involvement in evaluation is likely to produce results which are more relevant to the needs of communities than the needs of mental health agencies and that citizens will not have the same commitment to a particular programme or form of treatment as do in-house agency evaluators. Flaherty and Olsen (1978) found that compliance with the particular requirement to involve community residents in evaluation and quality assurance was very low.

Dinkel suggests seven major categories of evaluation activities in which citizens can play a part, with increasing degrees of citizen control:

> Citizens as subjects (community or client surveys)
> Citizens receive evaluation information through the media or at open forums
> Citizens act as a liaison between the community and the agency
> Citizens review programme goals
> Citizens review evaluation findings
> Citizens help plan agency evaluation
> Citizens conduct evaluation independently or with the agency

Mogulof (1974) believes there are three basic roles for citizen participation and that Federal policies are unclear about the specific role to be adopted by various Federal programmes. These roles are: advisory (transitional role where there is little decision-making power for citizens); adversary/control (either citizens or agency have real control while the other becomes adversarial to gain influence); coalition (decision-making is shared by citizens and agency).

Dinkel et al (1981) identify several barriers to citizen evaluation:

> Citizen board members are resistant to community citizens other than themselves being involved
> Centre staff resist sharing power with citizens
> There are few incentives for citizens to be involved and they are often unaware of the opportunities for them to participate or of the influence they have
> Citizens lack knowledge about the Centre and evaluation techniques
> The lack of back-up resources to support citizens limit their ability to work independently or follow-up their decisions

There is a lack of knowledge of demonstrated procedures for accomplishing citizen review.

On the basis of a survey of nine CMHC's, Flaherty and Olsen (1978), recommended the following actions to improve citizen participation in evaluation:

The specific goals of citizen involvement in evaluation should be identified

A definition of what is meant by "representative citizens" should be developed

The purposes of the annual reports and plans (produced by service providers) should be clarified by legislation and guidelines; (the UK white paper 'Caring for People' re quires this)

Reports and plans should be written to be understandable to lay citizens and should be disseminated to the public

The government should spell out proper channels for disseminating the reports and plans for quality assurance to those who should receive the information

Citizen boards should be informed of existing data about the operation of the service and these should be made available on an annual basis

Technical assistance to citizens could be done by increasing the dissemination of materials to various consumer/citizen groups.

We might add that special funds ought to be made available to groups charged with the responsibility for oversight of the quality of mental health programmes, to enable them to commission evaluative work in partnership with outside consultants who can provide them with the expert guidance which they lack in matters of monitoring and evaluation of services.

Summary and conclusions

1
The main stakeholders involved in the delivery of mental health services appear to be: the employees' managing agency; the professional body (or bodies) of which the employee is a member; the workers who share responsibility with an individual employee for the delivery of services; the people using services and their carers (usually families); the communities (or their representatives) within which services are delivered.

2
Ciarlo (1982) suggests that two types of programme accountability had tended to dominate CMHC programmes, the 'performance measurement' type at the federal and state level, and the 'quality assurance' type at the local level.

3
The professional body (or bodies) of which the employee is a member has traditionally been a fairly weak line of accountability for workers, although professional bodies have been involved with the setting of standards and the development of ethical codes.

4
The growth of the 'consumer movement' in mental health mirrored the general impact of consumerism in the United States during the 1960's and 1970's. Health care consumption is a very different form of consumerism from that of cash exchange for an industrially-manufactured product (Taylor 1983).

5
Administrators and mental health workers saw potential gains from client involvement in the mental health system and in the creation of alternative services. One author specified seven potential benefits: increased sense of client self-esteem; increased optimism about recovering; development of innovative programmes more responsive to the needs of clients; decreased cost; creation of a community-based force of advocates for improved mental health services; provision of services to under-served populations; improved public image of the mentally ill (Kopolow 1981).

6
Altman (1978) identified 11 policy areas with potential for resident participation in institutional settings. But involvement was not to be confined to institutional settings. The involvement of user and ex-user activists took several forms, including: input to agency policy and budget control; service provision by users themselves; systems of advocacy, advice and representation; surveys and evaluation studies involving people using services; education of planners and mental health workers; protest and pressure group activity; and litigation.

7
Client satisfaction scales were developed during the late 1970's and early 1980's (e.g. Essex et al 1981). Fisher (1983) has pointed out that satisfaction surveys have some serious drawbacks.

8
Colom (1981) argues that client representation can be obtained, but requires the active recruitment, orientation and training of clients in regard to the mental health and social service delivery systems to ensure informed participation as well as the training of clients to serve as advocates, self-advocates and members of boards.

9
Windle and Paschall (1981) found that between 1972 and 1979 the proportion of community mental health centres reporting use of a client complaints system rose from 10% to 48%.

10
Kaufmann et al (1979) reviewed over 80 client satisfaction surveys. Areas of general agreement included impact of treatment (91% felt that services had helped them), overall satisfaction (87% were satisfied), confidentiality (81% felt that it was important and 90% felt that the programme kept their problems confidential), and follow-up (86% would like their therapists to telephone them shortly after they stopped treatment).

11
Kopolow (1981) defines three major types of ex-patient operations. These are independent self-help, the collaborative programme and the advocacy programme.

12
Roman and Schmais (1972) have characterised the community boards which developed as a consequence of US Federal legislation, promoting community participation in a range of fields during the 1960's, under five general types according to their formal role. These are: the incorporated body model; the delegated authority model; the shared responsibility model; the issue delegation model; and the most common, the Purley Advisory model.

13
Riley (1981) suggests that community participation in service delivery can be made operational in at least three ways: the use of volunteers, the use of clients as service deliverers, and the employment of individuals identified with clients through cultural similarity and social activism on their behalf (paraprofessionals). Riley concludes that citizen participation in service delivery is poorly conceptualised, the greatest failure being lack of specific techniques by which it is to be achieved and cultivated.

14
Windle (1979) has gathered empirical evidence that having the public involved in evaluation or made aware of findings does increase the likelihood that the findings will be used. Dinkel et

al (1981) suggest that citizen involvement in evaluation is likely to produce results which are more relevant to the needs of communities than the needs of mental health agencies.

15

Dinkel et al (1981) identify several barriers to citizen evaluation: citizen board members are resistant to community citizens other than themselves being involved; centre staff resist sharing power with citizens'; there are few incentives for citizens to be involved and they are often unaware of the opportunities for them to participate or of the influence they have; citizens lack knowledge about the Centre and evaluation techniques; the lack of back-up resources to support citizens limits their ability to work independently or follow-up their decisions; and there is a lack of knowledge of demonstrated procedures for accomplishing citizen review.

References

Altman, R. et al (1978) Resident Participation in Institutional Policy. *Exceptional Children* 44(8):619-621.

Brandon, D. (1981) *Voices of Experience: Consumer Perspectives of Psychiatric Treatment.* MIND, London.

British Psychological Society (1986) *Responsibility Issues in Clinical Psychology and Multidisciplinary Community Teamwork.*

Chamberlin, J. (1979) *On Our Own: Patient-Controlled Alternatives to the Mental Health System.* Hawthorn Books, New York.

Chu, F. (1984) The Nader Report: One Author's Perspective. *Amer. Jnl. of Psychiatry* 131(7):7.

Ciarlo, J. (1982) Accountability Revisited: The Arrival of Client Outcome Evaluation. *Evaluation and Programme Planning* 5:31-36.

Colom, E. (1981) Reaction of an Angry Consumer. *Community Mental Health Journal* 17(1) Spring.

D.H.S.S. (1980) *Organisational and Management Problems of Mental Illness Hospitals.* HMSO, London.

Dinkel, N. et al (1981) Citizen Participation in C.M.H.C. Program Evaluation: A Neglected Potential. *Community Mental Health Journal* 17(1) Spring.

Dowell, D., and Ciarlo, J. (1983) Overview of the C.M.H.C. program from an evaluation perspective. *Community Mental Health Journal* 19(2) Summer.

Durlak, J. (1979) Comparative Effectiveness of Paraprofessional and Professional Helpers. *Psychological Bulletin* 86:80-92.

Essex, D. et al (1981) The Development, Factor Analysis, and Revision of a Client Satisfaction Form. *Community Mental Health Journal* 17(3):226-235.

Fisher, M. ed (1983) *Speaking of Clients.* Joint Unit for Social Services Research, University of Sheffield.

Flaherty, E. and Olsen, K. (1978) *An Assessment of the Utility of Federally required Program Evaluation in C.M.H.Cs.* Philadelphia Health Management Corporation (N.I.M.H. Contract No. 278-77-0067(MH)).

Glenn, R. (1975) Measuring patients' opinions about hospitalisation using the client satisfaction scale. *Hospital and Community Psychiatry* 26:15-16.

Kaufmann, S. et al (1979) Synthesising the Interests of Consumers, Citizens, and Administrators in Gathering Client Feedback. *Evaluation and Program Planning* 2:263-267.

Kopolow, L. (1981) Client Participation in Mental Health Service Delivery. *Community Mental Health Journal* 17(1) Spring.

Larsen, D. et al (1979) Assessment of Client/Patient Satisfaction: Development of a General Scale. *Evaluation and Program Planning* 2:197-207.

Lebow, (1982) Models for Evaluating Services at Community Mental Health Centres. *Hospital and Community Psychiatry* 33(12).

Love, R. et al (1979) The User Satisfaction Survey: Consumer Evaluation of an Inner City C.M.H.C. *Evaluation and the Health Professions* 2:42-54.

Mogulof, M. (1974) Advocates for Themselves: Citizen Participation in Federally Supported Community Organisations. *Community Mental Health Journal* 10(1):66-77.

Nassi, A. J. (1978) Community Control or Control of the Community? The Case of the C.M.H.C. *Jnl of Community Psychology* 6:3-15.

Overtveit, J. (1986) *Organisation of Multidisciplinary Community Teams*. Brunel Institute of Organisation and Social Studies, Middlesex, England.

Peck, E. (1986) *Consumerism and Mental Health Services.*Interdisciplinary Association of Mental Health Workers' Bulletin No. 6 November.

P.S.S.R.U. (1987) *Care in the Community Bulletin 7* Autumn University of Kent, Canterbury.

Reiff, R. and Riessman, F. (1965) The Indigenous Paraprofessional. *Community Mental Health Journal Monograph* No. 1.

Riley, W. (1981) Citizen Participation in C.M.H.C. Service Delivery. *Community Mental Health Journal* 17(1) Spring.

Riley, W. et al (1980) Paraprofessionals and Parapose: The Case of the Paraprofessional in the C.M.H.C. In S. Robin and M. Wagenfeld (eds) *Paraprofessionals in the Human Services*. Behavioral Publications, New York.

Roman, M., and Schmass, A. (1972) Consumer Participation and Control: A Conceptual Overview. In H. Barten and L. Bellak (eds) *Progress in Community Mental Health*. Grune and Stratton, New York.

Slater, V. et al (1982) A Satisfaction with Mental Health Care Scale. *Comprehensive Psychiatry* 23(1) Jan/Feb.

Social Services Committee 1984/85 Session (1985) Second Report, *Community Care with Special Reference to Adult Mentally Ill and Mentally Handicapped People*. HMSO, London.

Taylor, D. (1983) *The Consumer Movement, Health and the Pharmaceutical Industry*. Office of Health Economics,London.

Thomson, R. (1973) The Whys and Why Nots of Consumer Participation. *Community Mental Health Journal* 9(2).

Windle, C. (1979) The Citizen as Part of the Management Process.' In. H. Schulberg and J. Jerrell (eds) *The Evaluator and Management*. California, Sage Publications.

Windle, C., and Paschall, N. (1981) Client Participation in C.M.H.C. Program Evaluation: Increasing Incidence, Inadequate Involvement. *Community Mental Health Journal* 17(1) Spring.

173

7 Evaluation of services

Introduction

In this chapter we review papers and books which describe evaluation methods, the purposes of evaluation, monitoring and information systems, and other, less classifiable, aspects of evaluation. Given the confusion of purpose, and the willingness of professionals and others to 'project' their own view of purposes onto CMHCs (see the opening chapters), one can hardly be surprised that the literature on how to evaluate CMHCs is so wide-ranging, voluminous, and for the most part, inconclusive. We will again largely be concerned with the evaluation of services for identified mental health problems, although we will consider the role and performance of psychiatric screening for morbidity which would otherwise remain undetected. For the evaluation of preventive effort see the chapter on effectiveness.

Most of the work reviewed in the present chapter is 'data-free', that is, the authors, in expounding a view about the wisdom of one or other evaluative practices, do not (usually) provide their own supporting evidence. In the chapters on efficiency and effectiveness we have already reviewed the evidence which does exist, and we do not propose to repeat ourselves. We include the present chapter because, in the context of service developments in the UK, there is a growing desire for information about evaluation practice. Some of the sources we cite may prove useful to service planners, providers, and evaluators, in their attempts to justify innovation, expenditure and research. We have to say

that, on the whole, we are not impressed by the 'data-free' literature, but we are prepared to let others judge the quality, and the
value of the material, for their own purposes.

We would like to quote, and endorse, a pertinent remark,
attributed to Endicott, by Braun & Irving (1984):

> Poor program evaluation is counterproductive in many
> other ways than being a waste of money. It makes it
> doubly difficult to introduce good evaluation programs
> later because of staff attitude. It often produces mislead-
> ing results, and sometimes leads to unwarranted conclu-
> sions. The best kinds of program evaluation contrast
> alternative ways of delivering services to well defined
> target groups. Such evaluations can thus lead to decisions
> based upon good comparative cost-benefit data.

Evaluation reviews

Freeman & Solomon (1979) review the rapid growth of evaluation research, and observe that this process has been marked by:
the establishment of an 'entrepreneurial industry' of considerable proportions; the emergence of a new profession; the federal
recognition of the importance of evaluation; an increase in quality control effort; and attempts to solve methodological and
dissemination problems. A wealth of material has become available, leading to the creation of 'guides' for the prospective user
(Atkinson et al, 1979; Backer et al, 1980), and overviews of the
whole field (including research instruments) (e.g.Clark & Friedman, 1983; Coursey et al, 1977; Fox & Rappaport, 1972; Hagedorn
et al, 1976; Hargreaves et al, 1979; Schulberg & Bromet, 1981;
Stevenson & Longabaugh, 1980; Struening,1983).

Existing research evaluation has, in the opinion of some
reviewers 'done more to question the value of, rather than
improve the quality of' the services studied (Hersey,1979). There
is a good deal of difference between evaluation for practitioners
and for planners, and deciding who the evaluation is for, and who
should do it, are two of the central questions to address, before
the enterprise begins (Coursey, 1977; McIntyre, 1977; Specter,
1977). Mitchell (1977) usefully summarises some of the major
dimensions of evaluative work. He divides evaluation into studies
of: direct and indirect outcomes; program goal setting; social area
analysis; monitoring and information systems; fiscal monitoring;
and utilisation review (a term which is used technically, by
Goldblatt et al (1979) to mean a system of 'peer review').

In an intriguing paper, Siegel & Doty, (1978) contrast two
styles of evaluation, 'advocacy research', and 'management
review'. They use, as an example of the former (AR), the work of
Chu & Trotter (1974) and the US government's General Account-

ing Office (GAO) as an example of the latter (MR). (UK equivalents might be MIND and the Audit Commission!). They describe the differences between the two styles as: MR tends to accept the policymakers' basic assumptions about the goals of social policy, whereas AR questions the basis of this policy; MR tends to be done by Units which are subordinate to the policymakers, whereas AR tends to be independent; AR researchers court controversy in making their case, whereas MR tends to avoid it; MR tends to be rationalist and tries to pretend that policy does not exist, while AR tends to be Utopian, seeing political obstacles but regarding them as utterly illegitimate.

The occupational hazards of MR are a tendency to shrink back from the implications of controversial findings, and to avoid making policy recommendations except those which are not offensive. AR's occupational hazards are rhetorical posturing, overstatement and exaggeration, a search for sweeping panaceas and a tendency to look for villains and their invidious motivations, instead of structural factors and their remedies. They conclude:

> if used in combination, they complement each other quite effectively,...combining review of changes within the system and of the system, even if the proponents of each approach would not touch the others' method with a ten foot pole.

These two styles can be seen at work in existing mental health care policy and evaluation practice in the UK. There are very few places where a balanced approach combining the two styles can be found. Evaluators need to be independent, to a degree, but financial realities mean that research, particularly applied research of this sort, is funded mainly from government sources.

By the 1980s, some commentators were arguing the case for the central importance of client outcome studies (Ciarlo,1982; Schainblatt, 1980). Client outcome studies, which surely are the most important aspect of service evaluation, represent a 'significant move beyond' the two models most commonly in use - performance measurement and quality assurance (Ciarlo, 1982).

Performance measurement and quality assurance

There appears to have been relatively little useful output from the use of performance measurement and quality assurance programmes. Conceptual and operational problems abound, (Fernandez, 1979; Forstenzer, 1980; Porter, 1977) and it is not surprising that evaluators tend to fall back on client outcome measures as the best (and most useful) indicators. Connolly &

Deutsch (1980) point out that judging the performance of a service very much depends upon where the judge stands - there are 'multiple constituencies' who may not agree on the operational criteria for adequate performance . Etzioni (1960) argued that the competing sub-systems in an organisation made 'goal achievement' virtually impossible. In fact, he argued that organisations failed to achieve goals not because of poor planning, unanticipated consequences, or an hostile environment, but because they are not meant to be realised. For Etzioni, goals are cultural entities, or sets of meanings 'depicting target states'.

At a clinical level, rather than an organisational level, the same problems persist. Methods for assessing the level and quality of clinical care, depend very much on the person undertaking the assessment, and the subject of the assessment. Methods for correcting inadequate levels of care may be more easily defined than operated. Grant (1982) concludes that peer review (see also Brook & Appel, 1973; Riedel et al 1972) is the most appropriate process for assessing the quality of care in CMHCs.

Keppler-Seid et al (1980) suggest that performance measures will only improve service systems when they are accompanied by supportive research, which can provide an independent assessment of the performance, (and of the adequacy of the performance measures themselves, when judged against external criteria). Preparation for the use of performance indicators, wide participation, and the use of tested systems are all advocated by Keppler-Seid et al, if the system is to work successfully. An essential prerequisite is that existing systems are replaced, so that the new performance measures are not introduced on top of them, but as a replacement.

Some of the work which falls into the category of quality assurance can be called 'descriptive program evaluation'. The service, or a particular aspect of the service, for example, the 'atmosphere' on the ward are assessed and rated by observers. The best known examples of this type of performance measurement are the PASS (Program Analysis of Service Systems) system (Wolfensberger & Glenn, 1973), the Ward Atmosphere Scale (Moos, 1974), and the COPES (Community Oriented Programs Environment Scale) (Moos,1972). This approach has the advantage that outsiders are required to undertake the observations, but is heavily dependent upon the achievement of reliability in areas which require a good deal of subjective judgement.

Monitoring and management information systems

Wing's distinction (Wing & Hailey, 1972) between evaluation (which usually involves comparison) and monitoring (which involves the routine collection of information) is a useful one, which is maintained in the present report. Without regular collection of information about service use and provision, changes in use, which may occur in response to major policy decisions, resource changes, or social factors, cannot be studied. Morosini et al (1985) suggest that the major changes in Italy's services cannot be adequately evaluated because of the shortcomings of the Italian national information system (ISTAT).

In the USA the federal requirement for CMHCs to evaluate their activity (Feldman & Windle,1973; Flaherty & Windle,1981; Neigher et al, 1982; Windle,1979), under Law PL 90-174, and later PL 94-63, resulted in two approaches. First, there were funds from NIMH for specific studies, and second, independent evaluations following the federal guidelines. The CMHC was required to spend 2% of its operating costs on evaluation. Discussion of the '2% evaluation effort' can be found in Flaherty & Olsen (1982), Cook & Shadish (1982) and Landsberger et al (1979). Neigher et al confirm that, while evaluation technology might have improved as a result of this effort, there seems to be a general feeling that a co-ordinated and systematic approach was lacking. A major opportunity to study the impact of social policy was missed.

Flaherty & Windle (1981) suggest that the assumptions underlying Law 94-63, were only partly supported by evidence, and that the self-evaluation, citizen review, state standards, and technical assistance which resulted, were misguided, and the results disappointing. Windle (Flaherty & Windle, 1981; Windle, 1979) argues in favour of state funded research, but directed at the impact and effectiveness of services. As early as 1973 Feldman & Windle concluded that CMHCs were 'ill-equipped to develop evaluation programs of their own'. Nothing published subsequently suggests otherwise.

The lesson of the US and Italian experiences is that instead of requiring centres to evaluate themselves, they should be required to collect routine statistics, preferably with a standard core set of data and additions which reflect local circumstances. A percentage of the development monies for centres should be put aside for both the establishment and running of an information system, and for buying in outside evaluation. Unless this is done the mistakes of the US CMHC evaluation will simply be repeated.

In some cases the routine collection of information will extend to clinical records (Ciarlo,1977), and these may be used in outcome studies (Allen et al, 1980). Management information systems are only partly concerned with clinical records. Cooper (1979) suggests that they should also include information about the target population (from census data), the input of resources, staff activities and financial information. The design of such systems is itself the subject of a large literature (Chapman, 1976; Cooper, 1973;1979; Hollingshead, 1979; Siegel, 1980; Smith &

Sorensen, 1974). Atkinson & Nguyen (1981) have argued that the information required by management 'can be almost entirely derived from the information pool necessary for effective management of service delivery at the community based service level'.

For 'management purposes' the system must provide information that: defines how resources are being spent; determines the patterns of service delivery; provides monitoring aids for programme managers; provides data for multiple reporting requirements of funding agencies; and generates necessary data for planning purposes (Chapman, 1976). Considerable work has been done on data standards in the US mental health services, culminating in recommendations for a comprehensive system from the NIMH. Leginski et al (1989) divide the data required into five sets: patient\client data; event data; human resources data; financial data; and impact data.

Increasingly such information is held as a computerised record (Bloom, 1972; Crawford et al, 1974; Siegel & Goodman, 1976; Fagin & Purser, 1986). Fagin & Purser (1986) describe the system developed for the 608 CMHC in Waltham Forest, in London. 608 is based in a house in the community, uses a key worker system, and was intended to replace the hospital as 'the co-ordinating headquarters of mental health work outside the institution'. It was to be responsive to primary care referrals and provide a gateway to specialist services. The service was intended to be more accessible and friendly than the traditional psychiatric setting. The staff wanted to monitor referrals, largely to assess the impact of the new service. Large case registers (such as those at Salford and Nottingham) can monitor the use of services, and give an indication of levels of treated psychiatric morbidity; the 608 register was designed to cover a smaller geographical area, but to provide greater detail on individual cases.

The 608 register was to be sufficiently detailed to be useful to Centre workers, reliable (a manual was produced), capable of storing change data, provide quick access for routine administrative purposes and data for small scale evaluation projects. The assessment formulation was the core of the system. Each case record was made up of 120 data-fields, 42 of which could accept multiple values and so store longitudinal data. The results of using this system are not yet available.

The system does not, so far as we know enable cost data to be collected, except insofar as items of service are measured, which can be costed separately. A number of authors consider the type of cost information necessary in community mental health service provision (e.g Cooper, 1979; Newman et al, 1978).

Methods and techniques of evaluation

There are several evaluation models and each makes use of a

different range of techniques and methods. In the space available here we cannot hope to cover all of these, but we attempt to give an idea of the range of techniques which have been used.

Evaluation takes a number of forms , which for the sake of simplicity we can refer to as: outcome evaluation (of individual and group treatments for clients); goal directed evaluation (either of individuals, or of the service as a whole); fiscal evaluation; performance and quality evaluation; planning and management evaluation; and impact evaluation (including the impact on the community and the extent to which identified needs in the community are met).

For the most part outcome evaluation has been dealt with in the chapter on effectiveness, as has goal directed evaluation. Fiscal evaluation has been considered in the chapter on efficiency, and performance evaluation has been considered above. We will consider impact evaluation when we discuss needs assessment, and also at the end of this chapter in the section on miscellaneous aspects of evaluation. Management evaluation is also considered in the miscellaneous section.

First in the range of techniques to be discussed here, are outcome evaluation instruments. A number of these were developed in the USA to study the impact of CMHCs on clients. In the UK these tend to be divided into clinical and social assessments instruments. The use of these instruments has been widely reported, (e.g Ciarlo & Reihman, 1977; Wilson, 1977; Ellis et al, 1984) as have the results which they have produced (see Goldberg & Huxley, 1980), and the problems involved in their use (Effectiveness chapter above, and Platt, 1981).

The application of standard research interviews in an attempt to measure the impact of treatment is a commonly adopted approach. Case studies, participant observation (Glaser & Backer, 1973) and network analysis (Burgess et al, 1974) are less commonly adopted methods. Bickel & Forsyth-Stevens (1983) report on the use of case histories in the evaluation of community support programs, and Fry (1973) argues for the use of participant observation as a preliminary to more scientific approaches to evaluation. Huxley et al (1987) used an observational approach as an aid to the selection of appropriate evaluation methods. Frankel (1982) used participant observation in order to study the 'processes' at work in a therapeutic environment.

Network analysis (Engelberg, 1980) is a form of systems analysis which documents the client's contacts with agencies in a service system. Inferences are drawn from the total number of agencies contacted, the duplication of agencies, and the different patterns of agency contact. Bass & Windle (1972) report on attempts to measure the continuity of care given to a client, after they have entered into the mental health care system. In essence they measured the extent to which client histories were passed on between agencies, and the extent of joint work by agencies.

There are difficulties of interpretation with regard to the concept of continuity (for instance when is it desirable and when not), and with regard to the meaning of different patterns of client contact within an after care system (what factors contribute to the need for aftercare, and why should one pattern be preferred to another, and under what circumstances) . There is little evidence in the literature that these conceptual difficulties have been adequately addressed (see the chapter on coordination).

Needs assessment

Similar problems beset attempts to define and measure 'needs'. A specific 'needs assessment' literature has developed (see Brewin et al, 1987). We feel that this approach to evaluation has something to offer, in spite of the difficulties involved. It is, on the one hand related to social area analysis, and territorial needs indicators, and on the other hand shares something with the individual assessment characteristic of both clinical work and the use of standardised assessment instruments. In the USA Public Laws 89-749 and 93-641 called for programs to be tied to needs assessments. Zangwill (1977) examined all the department of Health and Welfare's programs which required needs assessment and found that none of them defined it. Only two said how often it should be carried out. Kimmel (1977) argued that concepts of need assessment were so broad that they could encompass any technique, and that the results of needs analysis were frequently left unused.

A major area of conceptual confusion lies in the failure to keep a distinction between definitions and concepts of needs assessment, and the means by which such assessments are to be achieved. It is possible to construct typologies of both concepts and methods.

Conceptual issues

Stewart (1979) shows that the assessment of need can be divided into three distinct entities - assessment of the deficit, assessment of the desire and assessment of the solution. Similarly, need can be divided into a condition, a want, a lack or anything that is felt to be needed. Bradshaw (1977) divides needs into four types - felt, comparative, expressed, and normative. Although Royse & Drude (1982) say that need is therefore without conceptual boundaries, it would appear that, so long as one is clear which type of need one is talking about, some conceptual clarity can be introduced into needs assessment.

For the present purpose we need to distinguish between needs as problems which exist for individuals,(leaving aside whether these have yet been felt or expressed in terms of service demand) and needs for services (which may or may not exist as demands). Choosing the means for measuring the extent of the problem, and choosing the means for providing a solution, involves value judgements about the types of needs which are eligible to be met, their priority order, criteria for eligibility to receive service, which additional services might be needed, and, if more than one is needed, the priority order of new service, or extended service provision.

A distinction can be drawn between types of need which exist but for which service is not provided, and types of need which exist in users of existing services. In the former case, these needs or problems might be defined by the sufferer, or by the service (felt versus normative need). The problem sufferers might choose to bring their problem to the notice of others (expressed need) or the service provider might choose to look for people in the community who have problems which are similar in severity and type to those of existing service users (comparative need). In the latter case (the needs of existing service users), the problems may be unmet and a case may exist for the alteration of existing services so that they are more responsive to these needs (unmet needs). Brewin et al (1987) define a need (when functioning falls below some minimum specified level, and this has been caused by remediable or potentially remediable circumstances) as 'met' when it attracts some at least partly effective intervention, and when no other intervention of greater potential effectiveness exists. 'Unmet' need, therefore, is defined as that which attracts 'only partly effective or no intervention, and when no other interventions of greater potential effectiveness exist'. Given the difficulty of distinguishing between an 'at least partly effective intervention' and an 'only partly effective intervention' it might be easier to confine concepts of unmet need to situations where problems have not met with any response.

According to this model need can only exist when there is an intervention which is appropriate and potentially effective, and this requires a considerable, and perhaps unattainable, degree of consensus about the availability and appropriateness of effective interventions. Patients' views influence the model only when the potential effectivenes of the intervention is assessed. Set in the context of service delivery and the development of social policies to address questions of need, this model appears to relegate all new service and policy developments to the realms of hypothesis or fantasy. People with very similar problems may be divided, on the basis of professional agreement concerning what is available and effective, into those for whom solutions are available and those for whom they are not. Instead of those with problems for which there is no solution having 'unmet needs', they have 'no needs' according to this model. Two people with 'financial problems', one of whom is eligible for a grant because of the fact that he has children, and one of whom is not, because he is childless would be treated differently. The first would have a 'need' for financial assistance, but the other would have no 'need'. Brewin et al say that the judgement of 'no need' does not vitiate the search for innovative services; it would perhaps have been preferable , particularly for the social aspects of need, had they used the term 'unmet need' and further subdivided it into services available and not available, or in existence and not in existence.

Attempts to enable people, whether they are users or providers of service, to say what services they ideally need, ie those services which do not currently exist, do not work very well (Cox et al, 1979; SSRG,1986). Clients cannot be expected to construct an ideal service out of their individual needs or wants, and professionals too have difficulty speculating about innovative service design.

Methodological issues

Warheit et al (1974) describe five methods of needs assessment: the key informant approach, the community forum approach, the rates-under-treatment approach, the survey approach and the social indicators approach. Royse & Drude reduce the number to three general approaches - impressionistic, community surveys and epidemiological approaches, and social indicators. They outline the main problems with each, which are - impressionistic methods may be unrepresentative, community surveys suffer from definitional and sampling problems, and social indicators are only indirect measures.

Impressionistic methods, such as the use of key informants in the community, the use of 'nominal groups' (e.g. workshops of selected individuals) and community forum approaches, are certainly subjective and may be representative. They could be used to corroborate a service approach which was devised using a more reliable method.

Community surveys are a methodological improvement, and the standardisation of techniques in this field, together with improvements in census data and statistical modelling techniques, remove some of the earlier objections to their use. We now have a much more clear idea of rates and types of psychiatric disorder found in the community (Goldberg & Huxley, 1980).

There has been a good deal of debate about the use of social indicators (see the chapter on efficiency) and discussion of their place in needs assessment (Cochran, 1979; Kamis,1979; Kimmel, 1977; Varenais, 1977; Zangwill, 1977). As in community survey approaches, modern methods of data collection, storage and analysis allow us to use a wider range of data in more sophisticated ways. The reliability of this data is crucial. Pollack et al (1968) and many others since have drawn attention to some of the deficiencies of census data. Social indicator data is probably of most value in relation to decisions about resource allocation, rather than in relation to the evaluation of the effect of services on rates of morbidity.

Siegel & Attkisson (1979) report three examples of the use of social indicators in practice. Bloom (1968) studied services in Pueblo, Colorado, using 42 census variables, and found higher rates of hospitalisation in the socially disadvantaged inner city census tracts. Socio-economic affluence was related to higher rates of hospitalisation for minor morbidity in middle class areas, and to higher rates of hospitalisation for severe morbidity in lower class areas. The work of Galle et al (1972) was used to develop an Index of Need in Los Angeles County. 15 variables from public health and census data were used. They were chosen on the basis of the most frequently mentioned indicators associated, in epidemiological studies, with the need for mental health services. The index ignores private facilities.

The NIMH has developed the Mental Health Demographic Profile System (MHDPS) (Goldsmith et al, 1975). Relative risk for mental health problems is determined for each census tract on the basis of census data, and compared with the volume of service in each. (Once again there are crucial decisions to be made, not only about the acceptable census data, but also about measures of service input.) MHDPS data are not used to justify the program, but as an internal aid to allocating resources.

Royse & Drude (1982) recommend that guidelines for conducting needs assessments should be established, and that standard instruments, which permit comparisons, should be used. They suggest that a research project should be undertaken to assess the value of the different methodological approaches in the same geographical area. Given the recent improvements in data gathering and analysis in this field we would argue that the social indicator approach, in conjunction with the information from community morbidity surveys and case registers, is probably preferable, so far as resource allocation is concerned, to the notion of a standard or normative provision of services.

Other aspects of evaluation

The remainder of the literature can be divided into four parts. A number of papers describe methodological issues which relate to evaluation practices. There are a large number of papers which are concerned with the basic questions which any evaluation raises, such as the costs, the organisation and the evaluation of the evaluation! The evaluation of special types or aspects of services is the third category. Finally a number of papers address the issue of the generalisation of the results of an evaluation.

Methodology

Evaluation methodologies in the community mental health field are no different from those used in other fields of health and social care (see for example Datta & Perloff, 1979 and Struening et al , 1983).The problems which beset evaluation in this field are also the same. Several papers address the issue of the relative merits of quantitative and qualitative methods; most conclude that using both can be advantageous (Bednarz, 1985; Ginsberg,1984; Heilman, 1980). Qualitative methods are recommended for the early 'hypothesis formulation' stage of evaluation, sometimes called the 'formative' stage. Quantitative methods are recommended for the later 'hypothesis testing' stage ('summative' evaluation).

The technical problems of measuring change have also been considered in relation to mental health services (Dush,1983) and the issues here are no different from those in other fields (Nunnally, 1983; Tuchfeld, 1979). Ellsworth (1979) considers the effect of low response rates on the validity of evaluation results. He found no evidence to support the view that non-responders are different to responders in a postal survey concerned with the effectiveness of community mental health services.

Basic tasks and questions

A large literature is devoted to the tasks involved in selecting an appropriate method of evaluation, defining its purposes and calculating its costs. McIntyre (1977) and Coursey (1977) describe the basic tasks involved in setting up an evaluation, and Bunker (1978) considers how to organise an evaluation to serve the needs of managers and planners. Others have discussed the type of evaluation (e.g 'outcome evaluation' (Hargreaves et al , 1979); 'impact evaluation' (Allen & Sears, 1979; Boruch & Gomez, 1979)) , whether it should be conducted by outsiders, or by peers (Goldblatt et al, 1979; Specter, 1977; Strasser & Deniston, 1978), and its impact on management (Bigelow,1975)and practitioners (Mikawa, 1975; Rosenfield & Orlensky, 1961).

The extent to which staff should be involved in the design and execution of the evaluation, and how they are informed about the results are the subjects of papers by Friedman (1977) and Murrell (1977). Murrell also considers how to involve consumers, and Weiss et al (1977) look at citizen evaluation, while Hoshall & Friedman (1975) give a patient's view of evaluation. Abt (1979) and Seidenberg et al (1979) both consider the costs involved in an evaluation, and Windle (1977) the resources which are needed to conduct one.

A number of authors discuss the evaluation of very specific types of service. These include the evaluation of: community action programs (Brophy et al, 1977); statewide services (Berren,

1984); conferences (Canfield & Kliewer, 1979); hotlines (Genther, 1974); education and training programs (Goldstein, 1977; Guttentag et al, 1975); indirect services (Montague & Taylor, 1971); consultation (Cytrynbaum, 1977); and therapeutic communities (Berg,1979). Murrell & Brown (1977) discuss 'the evaluation of the evaluation'.

These papers represent a 'cookbook' approach, and their value is limited by the fact that they do not present any data about the results of having tried the approach, and they are highly context specific. A small number of papers describe the problems in generalising the results of evaluations, and these may be more useful. They enable us to think about the issues involved in dissemination and implementation of results before we undertake the evaluation.

Although the under-use and indeed the mis-use of evaluation results is well known (Rich, 1979), less is reported, about the use of results. Caplan (1976) attempted to identify what social science information was used, by whom, and for what purposes. He interviewed 204 US government officials, and found that 75% had used specific findings. Over half of the findings used were from program evaluations, and over half of these were on policy issues of national importance. Connolly & Porter (1980) point out that in 86% of the cases where findings were used, the user agency funded the project. The more important the policy area, the greater was the tendency to evaluate it internally to the agency. In 80% of cases the information used resulted from the specific request of a major 'decisionmaker' in the agency. One third of all used information was directed towards policy issues relating to the internal workings of the agency. They conclude that use is much more likely if findings are generated as a specific response to a policymaker's request.

The same authors cite some of the common reasons for the failure to use evaluation findings. These include: methodological weaknesses in the research; lack of attention to the policymaking timescale; the poor 'organizational placement' of the evaluation unit; the political naivete of evaluators; and the poor presentation and dissemination of findings. The last of these, poor dissemination, is widely held to be responsible for the non use of results (Weiss,1979; Hugman & Huxley, 1987). Better 'packaging' of results, advertising, styling (eliminating jargon) and market segmentation (targeting different versions of the same results to different audiences) have all been recommended as potentially useful in improving dissemination.

Another major contributory factor in the low use of evaluation results is the lack of relevance of the results. Connolly & Porter suggest that use is higher if the research is commissioned by a senior policymaker in an agency, since this presumably enhances the relevance of the findings. It is important to avoid what Mitroff & Featheringham (1974) call 'errors of the third kind'. An error of the third kind occurs when the evaluator provides a precise answer to the wrong question. Knowing the right question, or perhaps being able to distinguish between several 'right questions' in terms of their relevance and utility to service planners and providers, is an art form Very little attention has been paid to this ability (Hugman & Huxley, 1987).

In order for his/her results to be used in an appropriate way the evaluator needs to think about potential use, before and not after, the evaluation takes place. In a study of ten evaluations (seven funded by the NIMH) Weiss (1979) concludes that "when the evaluation was developed with no clear concept of who was to use the results, the report often wound up in no man's land". Smith & Caulley (1979) point out that this may be difficult to achieve when the nature of the service under evaluation changes while it is being evaluated. It may be extended beyond its original focus, become relevant to a new client group, or redefined because of external influences.

Sinclair (Marks et al, 1988) points out that there are three reasons why it is rare for a single piece of research to offer answers to a policy problem. First, the results ar usually less salient by the time the research is complete. Second, all researchers have 'angles' and all studies have defects, so several studies are needed before firm conclusions can be drawn. Third, policy problems usually involve more variables than are used in the research.

To some extent evaluators are still inclined to take a rational approach to the use of their results, assuming that utilisation will follow the presentation of relevant, timely, commissioned and 'consumable' reports. Bulmer (1982) and Weiss (1980) both suggest that research is not commissioned by policymakers with the intention of solving a specific problem. Policymakers use research in social policy making to orient themselves to problems. Janowitz (1972) said that the contribution of research was to create the intellectual conditions for problem solving.

Rich (1979) suggests that evaluators should concentrate more attention on the quality of utilisation, whether misuse occurs, and studying the process of use within bureaucratic organisations. Bachrach (1980) examines the problems of using results from model programs for chronic patients in other contexts. She points out that most model programs receive separate (and more adequate) funding, and that attempts to translate findings from experimental programs in to 'normal' services are handicapped by this and several other 'transfer' problems. These include, the ability of the model programme to be selective, to focus on clients whose chances of improvement are considerable, to draw boundaries around its main task, and to concentrate a greater proportion of its resources on evaluation.

187

References

Abt, C.C. (1979) Government Constraints on Evaluation Quality. In L.Datta & R.Perloff (1979) *Improving Evaluations.* Sage, New York.

Allen, H.M. & Sears, D.O. (1979) Against them or for me: Community Impact Evaluations. In L.Datta & R.Perloff (1979) *Improving Evaluations.* Sage, New York.

Allen, R.H., Webb, L.J. & Gold, R.S. (1980) Validity of Problem-oriented Record System for evaluating Treatment Outcome. *Psychological Reports* 47:303-306.

Atkinson, C.C. & Nguyen, T.D. (1981) Evaluative Research and Health Policy: Utility, Issues, and Trends. *Health Policy Quarterly* 1(1):22-41.

Attkisson, C.C., Hargreaves, W.A., Tuller, I.R., Temoshok, L., McIntyre, M.H. & Siegel, L.M. (1979) *A Workingpeople's Guide to The Community Mental Health Program Evaluation Literature.* In W.Hargreaves (ed) Resource Materials for CMH Program Evaluation. NIMH.

Bachrach, L. (1980) Overview: model programs for chronic mental patients. *Am.J. Psychiat.* 137(9):1023-1031.

Backer, T.E., Attkisson, C.C., Barry, J.R., Brock, T.C., Davis,H.R., Kiresuk, T.J., Kirkhart, K.E., Perloff, R. & Windle,C.(1980) Information Resources for Program Evaluators. *Evaluation & Program Planning* 3:22-33.

Bass, R.D. & Windle, C. (1972) Continuity of Care: An Approach to Measurement. *Am.J.Psychiat.* 129(2):196-201.

Bednarz, D. (1985) Quantity and Quality in Evaluation Research: A Divergent View. *Evaluation & Program Planning* 8:289-306.

Berg, W.E. (1979) The evaluation of treatment in therapeutic communities: Problems of design and implementation. *Evaluation & Program Planning* 2:41-48.

Berren, M.R. (1984) Statewide Outcome Evaluation: An Introduction to the Special Issue. *Community Mental Health Journal* 20(1):4-13.

Bickel, R. & Forsyth-Stevens, A. (1983) Using Case Histories in an Evaluation of Community Support Programs. *Psychosocial Rehabilitation Journal* VII(1):11-21.

Bigelow, D.A. (1975) The Impact of Therapeutic Effectiveness Data on Community Mental Health Center Management: The Systems Evaluation Project. *Community Mental Health Journal* 11(1):64-74.

Bloom, B.L. (1968) An Ecological Analysis of Psychiatric Hospitalisation. *Multivariate Behavioural Research* 1:307-320.

Bloom, B.L. (1972) Human accountability in a community mental health center: Report of an automated system. *Community Mental Health Journal* 8:251-260.

Boruch, R.F. & Gomez, H. (1979) Measuring Impact: Power Theory in Social Program Evaluation. In L.Datta & R.Perloff

(1979) *Improving Evaluations*. Sage, New York.

Bradshaw, J. (1977) The concept of social need. In N.Gilbert & H.Specht (eds) *Planning for Social Welfare*: Issues, models and tasks. Englewood Cliffs, Prentice Hall, New Jersey.

Braun, S.H. & Irving, D. (1984) A Natural History of Behavioural Health Program evaluation in Arizona. *Community Mental Health Journal* 20(1):56-71.

Brewin, C.R., Wing, J.K., Mangen, S.P., Brugha, T.S. & MacCarthy, B. (1987) Principles and practice of measuring needs in the long-term mentally ill: the MRC needs for care assessment. *Psychol. Med. 17.* (in press).

Brook, R.H. & Appel, F.A. (1973) Quality of Care Assessment: Choosing a Method for Peer Review. *New England Journal of Medicine* 288:1323-1329.

Brophy, M.C., Maisto, S., Burstein, L. & Chan, A. (1977) Evaluation of Community Action Programs: Issues and an Alternative. In Coursey R.D. (ed) *Program Evaluation for Mental Health*. Grune & Stratton, New York.

Bulmer, M. (1982) *The Uses of Social Research*. London, George Allen & Unwin.

Bunker, D.R. (1978) Organizing evaluation to serve the needs of program planners and managers. *Evaluation & Program Planning* 1:129-134.

Burgess, J., Nelson, R. & Wallhaus, R. (1974) Network analysis as a method for the evaluation of service delivery systems. *Community Mental Health Journal* 10: 337-344.

Canfield, M. & Kliewer, D. (1979) Conference Evaluation Manual. In Hargreaves, W.A., & Atkisson, C.C. (eds) (1979) *Resource materials for use in community mental health program evaluation*. DHEW Publication No.(ADM) 79-328, NIMH, Rockville, MD.

Caplan, N.(1976) Social Research and National Policy. *International Social Science Journal* 28.

Chapman, R.L. (1976) Statistical Subsystems II: Preliminary System Design. In Chapman, R.L. *The Design of Management Information Systems for Mental Health Organisations: A Primer*. NIMH, Rockville MD.

Chu, F. & Trotter, S. (1974) *The Madness Establishment*: Ralph Nader's Study Group Report on the NIMH. Grossman, New York.

Ciarlo, J.A. (1977) Monitoring and Analysis of Mental Health Program Outcome Data. *Evaluation* 4:109-114.

Ciarlo, J.A. (1982) Accountability Revisited: The Arrival of Client Outcome Evaluation. *Evaluation & Program Planning* 5:31-36.

Ciarlo, J.A. & Reihman, J. (1977) The Denver Community Mental Health Questionnaire: Development of a Multidimensional Program Evaluation Instrument. In Coursey R.D. (ed) *Program Evaluation for Mental Health*. Grune & Stratton, NY.

Clark, A. & Friedman, M.J. (1983) Nine standardised scales for evaluating treatment outcome in a mental health clinic. *J.Clin.Psychol.* 39(6):939-950.

Cochran, N. (1979) On the limiting properties of social indicators. *Evaluation & Program Planning* 2:1-4.

Connolly, T.C. & Deutsch, S.J. (1980) Performance Measurement: Some Conceptual Issues. *Evaluation & Program Planning* 3:35-43.

Connolly, T. & Porter, A.L. (1980) A User-Focused Model for the Utilization of Evaluation. *Evaluation & Program Planning* 3:131-140.

Cook, T.D. & Shadish, W.R. (1982) Metaevaluation: An assessment of the congressionally mandated evaluation system for community mental health centers. In G.J.Stahler & W.R.Tash. *Innovative Approaches to mental health evaluation.* Academic Press, New York.

Cooper, E.M. (1973) *Guidelines for a Minimal Statistical and Accounting System for Community Mental Health Services.* DHEW Publication No. (ADM) 74-14. NIMH, Rockville, MD.

Cooper, E.M. (1979) Essential Elements. In Hargreaves, W.A. (ed) *op cit.*

Coursey, R.D. (1977) Basic Questions and Tasks. In Coursey, R.D. (ed) (1977) *Program Evaluation for Mental Health.* Grune & Stratton, New York.

Coursey, R.D. (ed) (1977) *Program Evaluation for Mental Health.* Grune & Stratton, New York.

Cox, G.B., Carmichael, S.J. & Dightman, C.R. (1979) The Optimal Treatment Approach to Needs Assessment. *Evaluation & Program Planning* 2:269-275.

Crawford, G.L., Morgan, D.W. & Gianturco, D.T.(eds) (1974) *Progress in mental health information systems: Computer Applications.* Ballinger, Cambridge, Mass.

Cytrynbaum, S. (1977) The Review and Evaluation of Consultation Activities in a Community Mental Health Center: Some Pitfalls and Possibilities. In Coursey, R.D. (ed) (1977) *Program Evaluation for Mental Health.* Grune & Stratton, New York.

Datta, L. & Perloff, R. (1979) *Improving Evaluations.* Sage, New York.

Dush, D.M. (1983) Standardizing Outcome Data in Program Evaluation. *Community Mental Health Journal* 19(1):77-82.

Ellis, R.H., Wilson, N.Z. & Foster, F.M. (1984) Statewide Treatment Outcome Assessment in Colorado: The Colorado Client Assessment Record (CCAR). *Community Mental Health Journal* 20(1): 72-89.

Ellsworth, R.B. (1979) Does Follow-up Loss Reflect Poor Outcome? *Evaluation & the Health Professions* 2(4):419-437.

Engelberg, S.(1980) Network Analysis in Evaluation: Some Words of Caution. *Evaluation & Program Planning* 3:15-23.

Etzioni, A. (1960) Two Approaches to Organizational Analysis: A Critique and a Suggestion. *Administrative Science Quarterly* 5:257-278.

Fagin, L. & Purser, H. (1986) Development of the Waltham Forest Local Mental Health Case Register. *Bulletin of the Royal College of Psychiatrists* 10:303-306.

Feldman, S. & Windle, C. (1973) The NIMH Approach to Evaluating the Community Mental Health Centers Program. *Health Service Reports* 88(2):174-180.

Fernandez, D. (1979) Post Hoc Procedures fro Planning and Evaluation. *Evaluation & Program Planning* 2:219-222.

Flaherty, E.W. & Olsen, K. (1982) Impact of federally mandated program evaluation. *Community Mental Health Journal* 18(10:56-71.

Flaherty, E.W. & Windle, C. (1981) Mandated Evaluation in Community Mental Health Centers: Framework for a New Policy. *Evaluation Review* 5(5):620-638.

Forstenzer, H.M. (1980) Planning and Evaluation of Community Mental Health Programs. *Psychiatric Quarterly* 52(1):39-51.

Fox, P.D. & Rappaport, M. (1972) Some approaches to evaluating community mental health services. *Arch.Gen.Psychiat.* 26:172-178.

Frankel, B. (1982) On Participant Observation as a Component of Evaluation. *Evaluation & Program Planning* 5:239-246.

Freeman, H.E. & Solomon, M.A. (1979) The next decade in evaluation research. *Evaluation & Program Planning* 2:255-262.

Fry, L.J. (1973) Participant Observation and Program Evaluation. *J.Health & Soc. Behav.* 14:274-276.

Galle, O.R., Gove, W.R. & McPherson, J.M. (1972) Population density and pathology. *Science* 176:23-30.

Genther, R. (1974) Evaluating the Functioning of Community-Based Hotlines. *Professional Psychology* 5:409-414.

Ginsberg, P.E. (1984) The Dysfunctional Side Effects of Quantitative Indicator Production: Illustrations from Mental Health Care (A Message from Chicken Little). *Evaluation & Program Planning* 7:1-12.

Glaser, E.M. & Backer, T.E. (1973) A look at participant observation. *Evaluation* 1(3):46-49.

Goldberg, D.P. & Huxley, P.J. (1980) *Mental Illness in the Community: The Pathway to Psychiatric Care.* Tavistock, London.

Goldblatt, P.B., Henisz, J.E. & Tischler, G.L. (1979) Utilization Review Within an Institutional Context. In Hargreaves W.A. (ed) *op cit.*

Goldsmith, H.F., Unger, E.L., Rosen, B.M., Shambaugh, B.M. & Windle ,C. (1975) *A typological approach to doing sociological area analysis.* NIMH, Rockville MD.

Goldstein, I.L. (1977) Evaluation of Educational and Training Programs. In Coursey R.D. (ed) *Program Evaluation for Mental Health.* New York, Grune & Stratton.

Grant, R.L. (1982) Quality Assurance in Community Mental Health Centers: Why it may not be working. *Quality Review Bulletin* 8(9):3-7

Guttentag, M., Kiresuk, T., Oglesby, M. & Cann, J. (1975) *The evaluation of training in mental health.* Behavioral Publications.

Hagedorn, H.J., Beck, K.J., Neubert, S.F. & Werlin, S.H. (1976) *A working manual of simple program evaluation techniques for community mental health centers.* DHEW Publication No. (ADM) 76-404. NIMH, Rockville, MD.

Hargreaves, W.A. & Atkisson, C.C. (1979) Outcome studies in mental health program evaluation. In Hargreaves, W.A., & Atkisson, C.C. (eds) (1979) *Resource materials for use in community mental health program evaluation.* DHEW Publication No.(ADM) 79-328 NIMH, Rockville, MD.

Hargreaves, W.A., & Atkisson, C.C. (eds) (1979) *Resource materials for use in community mental health program evaluation.* DHEW Publication No.(ADM) 79-328 NIMH, Rockville, MD.

Heilman, J.G. (1980) Paradigmatic Choices in Evaluation Methodology. *Evaluation Review* 4(5):693-712.

Hersey, J.C. (1979) "Dirty" research in "real" places: A practitioner's guide to program evaluation in the human services. *Evaluation & Program Planning* 2:153-157.

Hollingshead, A.B. (1979) Monitoring Community Mental Health Services: A Case in Point. *Research in Community & Mental Health* 1:337-355.

Hoshall, D. & Friedman, J. (1975) Evaluation from a Former Patient's Point of View. *Evaluation* 2(2):8-9.

Hugman, R. & Huxley, P.J. (eds) (1987) *Working together: Research, Practice and Education in Social Work.* University of Lancaster, Lancaster.

Huxley, P.J., Korer, J., Jacob, C. & Hagan, T. (1987) *Evaluating Community Mental Health Services.* Manchester University, Mental Health Social Work Research Unit.

Janowitz, M. (1972) *Sociological Models and Social Policy.* General Learning Systems, New Jersey.

Kamis, E. (1979) A Witness for the Defense of Need Assessment. *Evaluation & Program Planning* 2:7-12.

Keppler-Seid, H., Windle, C. & Woy, J.R. (1980) Performance Measures for Mental Health Programs: Something Better, Something Worse, or More of the Same? *Community Mental Health Journal* 16(3):217-234.

Kimmel, W. (1977) *Needs Assessment: A Critical Perspective.* DHEW, Washington D.C.

Klerman, G. (1974) Current Evaluation Research on Mental Health Services. *Am.J.Psychiat.* 131(7):783-787.

Landsberger, G., Neigher, W.D., Hammer, R.J., Windle, C. & Woy, J.R. (eds) *Evaluation in Practice: A sourcebook of program evaluation studies from mental health care systems in the United States*. DHEW Publication N. (ADM) 78-763. Washington D.C.

Leginsky, W.A., Croze, C., Driggers, J., Dumpman, S., Geertsen, D., Kamis-Gould, E., Namerow, M.J., Patton, R.E., Wilson, Z. & Wurster, C. (1989) *Data standards for mental health decision support systems*. (ADM)89-1589 NIMH, Rockville, MD.

McIntyre, M. (1977) Approaching Program Evaluation: Clarifying Tasks. In Coursey, R.D. (ed) *op cit.*

Mikawa, J.K. (1975) Evaluations in community mental health. In P. McReynolds (Ed) *Advances in Psychological Assessment* (Vol.3) Jossey Bass, San Francisco.

Mitchell, N.L. (1977) A Suggested Schema for Utilization Review for a community mental health center. *J.National Med. Assoc.* 69(4):237-239.

Mitchell, R. (1977) The dimensions of an Evaluation System for Community Mental Health Centers. In Coursey R.D. (ed) *Program Evaluation for Mental Health*. Grune & Stratton, New York.

Mitroff, I.I. & Featheringham, T.R. (1974) On systematic problem solving and the error of the third kind. *Behavioral Science* 19:383-393.

Montague, E.K. & Taylor, E.N. (1971) *Handbook on Procedures for Evaluating Mental Health Indirect Service Programs in Schools*. Human Resources Research Organization, Alexandria, Virginia.

Moos, R. (1972) Assessment of the psychosocial environments of community-oriented psychiatric treatment programs. *Journal of Abnormal Psychology* 79:9-18.

Moos, R. (1974) *Evaluating treatment environments: A social ecological approach*. Wiley, New York.

Morosini, P.L., Repetto, F., De Salvia, D. & Cecere, F. (1985) Psychiatric Hospitalization in Italy Before and After 1978. *Acta Psychiat. Scand. Suppl* 316:27-43.

Murrell, S. (1977) Conducting a Program Evaluation: Collaboration, Feedback, and Open-System Perspectives. In Coursey R.D. (ed) *Program Evaluation for Mental Health*. Grune & Stratton, New York.

Murrell, S. & Brown, F. (1977) Judging Program Evaluations: Criteria in Contexts. In Coursey R.D. (ed) *Program Evaluation for Mental Health*. New York, Grune & Stratton.

Neigher, W., Ciarlo, J., Hoven, C., Kirkhart, K., Landsberg, G., Light, E., Newman, F., Struening, E.L., Williams, L., Windle, C., & Woy, J.R. (1982) Evaluation in the Community Mental Health Centers: A Bold New Approach? *Evaluation & Program Planning* 5:283-311.

Newman, F.L., Burwell, B.A. & Underhill, W.R. (1978) Program Analysis Using the Client Oriented Cost Outcome System. *Evaluation & Program Planning* 1:19-30.

Nunnally, J.C. (1983) The study of change in Evaluation research. In Struening E.L. Handbook of Evaluation Research. *op cit.*

Platt, S. (1981) Social Adjustment as a Criterion of Treatment Success: Just What Are We Measuring? *Psychiatry* 44(2):95-111.

Pollack, E.S., Redick, R.W. & Taube, C.A. (1968) The application of census socioeconomic and familial data to the study of morbidity from mental disorders. *Am.J.Pub.Health* 58:83-89.

Porter, W.H. (1977) A management by objectives approach to program evaluation. in Coursey R.D. (ed) *op cit.*

Reihman, J. & Ciarlo, J.A. (1979) A method for obtaining follow-up outcome data. In Hargreaves, W.A., & Atkisson, C.C. (eds) (1979) *Resource materials for use in community mental health program evaluation.* DHEW Publication No.(ADM) 79-328 NIMH, Rockville, MD.

Rich, R.F. (1979) Emerging Issues for Evaluators and Evaluation Users. In L.Datta & R.Perloff (1979) *Improving Evaluations.* Sage, New York.

Riedel, D.C., Brenner, M.H., Braver, L. Goldblatt, P., Klerman,G., Myers, J., Schwartz, C. & Tischler, G. (1972) Psychiatric utilization review as patient care evaluation. *Am. J. Pub Health* 62:1222-1228.

Rosenfield, J.M. & Orlensky, N. (1961) The effect of research on practice: Research and decrease of non continuance. *Arch. Gen.Psychiat.* 5:176-182.

Royal College of Psychiatrists (1987) *A Carer's Perspective.* R.C.of P., London.

Royse, D. & Drude, K. (1982) Mental Health Needs Assessment: Beware of False Promises. *Community Mental Health Journal* 18(2):97-106.

Schainblatt, A.H. (1980) What happens to the Clients. *Community Mental Health Journal* 16(4):331-342.

Schulberg, H.C. & Bromet, E. (1981) Strategies for Evaluating the Outcome of Community Services for the Chronically Mentally Ill. *Am. J.Psychiat.* 138(7):930-935.

Seidenberg, G.R. & Johnson, F.S. (1979) A Case Study in Defining Developmental Costs for Quality Assurance in Mental Health Center Programs. *Evaluation & Program Planning* 2:143-152.

Siegel, C. & Goodman, A.B. (1976) An Evaluative Paradigm for Community Mental Health Centers Using an Automated Data System. *Community Mental Health Journal* 12(2):215-227.

Siegel, J.M. (1980) Automated management information systems. *Admin. in Mental Health* 8(1):46-55.

Siegel. K. & Doty, P. (1978) "Advocacy Research" versus "Management Review": Nader's Raiders and G.A.O. on Community Mental Health Centers. *International Journal of Comparative Sociology* XIX(1-2):139-167.

Siegel, L.M. & Attkisson, C.C. (19790 Mental Health Needs Assessment: Strategies and Techniques. In Hargreaves, W.A., & Attkisson, C.C. (eds) (1979) *Resource materials for use in community mental health program evaluation*. DHEW Publication No.(ADM) 79-328 NIMH, Rockville, MD.

Smith, N.L. & Caulley, D.N. (1979) Post evaluation determination of a program's generalizability. *Evaluation & Program Planning* 2:297-302.

Smith, T.S. & Sorensen, J.E. (eds) *Integrated Management Information Systems for Community Mental Health Centers*. DHEW Publication No. (ADM) 75-165 NIMH, Rockville, MD.

Social Services Research Group (SSRG) (1986) *Monitoring the Mental Health Act*. Birmingham University.

Specter, G.A. (1977) The uses and abuses of the outside evaluator. In Coursey R.D. (ed) *op cit.*

Stevenson, J.F. & Longabaugh, R.H. (1980) The Role of Evaluation in Mental Health. *Evaluation Review* 4(4):461-479.

Stewart, R. (1979) The Nature of Needs Assessment in Community Mental Health. *Community Mental Health Journal* 15(4):287-295.

Strasser, S. & Deniston, O.L. (1978) Pre- and post-planned evaluation: which is preferable? *Evaluation & Program Planning* 1:195-202.

Struening, E.L. (1983) *Handbook of Evaluation Research*. Sage, New York.

Tuchfield, B.S. (1979) Some approaches to assessing change. In Datta & Perloff (eds) *op cit.*

Varenais, K. (1977) *Needs Assessment: An Exploratory Critique*. DHEW Washington D.C.

Warheit, G.J., Bell, R.A., & Schwab, J.J. (1974) *Planning for Change: Needs Assessment Approaches*. NIMH, Rockville, MD.

Weiss, C. (ed) (1980) *Social Science Research & Decision Making*. Columbia University Press, New York.

Weiss, C. (1979) Between the cup and the lip. In Hargreaves, W.A., & Atkisson, C.C. (eds) (1979) *Resource materials for use in community mental health program evaluation*. DHEW Publication No.(ADM) 79-328 NIMH, Rockville, MD.

Weiss, C., Monroe, J., Bray, C., Davis, H. & Hunt, B. (1977) Evaluation by Citizens. In Coursey R.D. (ed) *Program Evaluation for Mental Health*. Grune & Stratton, New York.

Wilson, N.C. (1977) The Automated Tri-Informant Goal Oriented Note: One Approach to Program Evaluation. In Coursey R.D. (ed) *Program Evaluation for Mental Health*. Grune & Stratton, New York.

Windle, C. (1977) Resources to Aid Mental Health Program Evaluation. In Coursey R.D. (ed) *Program Evaluation for Mental Health*. Grune & Stratton, New York.

Windle, C. (1979) Developmental Trends in Program Evaluation. *Evaluation & Program Planning* 2:193-196.

Wing, J.K. & Hailey, A. (1972) *Evaluating a Community Psychiatric Service*. Oxford, OUP.

Wolfensberger, W. & Glenn, L. (1973) *Program Analysis of Service Systems Handbook*. National Institute on Mental Retardation, Toronto.

Zangwill, B. (1977) *A compendium of laws and regulations requiring needs assessment*. DHEW, Washington D.C.

8 Key items in the development of effective services

Introduction

In this chapter we look in more detail at two of the key items in the development of effective community services for mentally ill people. These items have been referred to above, but are elaborated upon in this chapter. First, coordinated and efficient services seem to be associated with greater benefit to clients, in particular those with long-term problems. A major contribution could be made here by the use of case management. Second, as the resourcing of service in the UK becomes more and more mixed, and more like the US system the contribution of devolved budgets and the assessment of the quality of life assume more importance. The chapter ends with a small number of general conclusions and recommendations.

Case management

An important development in the provision of a coordinated service, and one which makes use of thorough assessment procedures combined with the amalgamation of resources from several agents, is the concept of 'case management'. There have been a number of papers reporting the use of this system in relation to elderly and mentally ill people (see coordination chapter). Its proponents regard it as particularly suited to providing care in the community for people with long-term problems.

It is widely used in the USA. A recent bibliography (GAO, 1988) identified 109 literature citations for case management as applied in the social services field, and 9 citations for agency/client contracting as applied to the delivery and receipt of such services. Case management is widely used in the care of elderly people (Morris, 1987; Seltzer, 1987), and has been used in child care services (Garrison, 1986; McDaniel, 1986; Wagner, 1987) and in mental health services (Raschko, 1985; Baier, 1987; Dickey et al , 1986; Franklin et al, 1987; Harris & Bergman, 1987; Intagliata & Baker, 1983; Wright et al, 1987; Marlowe, 1983; Wilson, 1983).

In case management, care is provided through the individually planned combination of different sources of support, and the whole care package may be overseen by a single 'case manager'. It is possible to combine private, voluntary and statutory sectors of care. In some examples of the approach the budget is also administered by the case manager. Individual assessment is emphasised and an attempt is made to meet the needs revealed, and to avoid simply fitting the client into the existing service system.

Austin & Greenberg (1984) point out that case management has become a core component in the delivery of long term care services. It is widely viewed as a mechanism for linking and coordinating segments of a service delivery system (within a single agency or involving several providers) to ensure the most comprehensive program for meeting an individual client's needs for care. Although there is some consensus regarding generic case management functions, the role of case manager is implemented with considerable variation and has different meanings in various settings (see also Bachrach, 1983). Austin (1981) argues that case management as implemented in programs for the elderly, has focused on interactions between the client and case manager in the areas of assessment, care planning, service plan implementation, and follow-up, and points out that variation in these case management tasks suggests that no single model can be implemented in all local delivery systems. Furthermore, she believes that:

> this emphasis on client/case manager interaction has obscured the fact that care planning, a core case management task, is a crucial resource allocation activity and has important consequences for the distribution of resources within a local delivery system. A resource dependence view of interorganizational relationships is useful for analysing the capacity of case managers to change market conditions by altering service providers' behaviour. The extent of discretion over resource allocation and centralisation of resource control are key case management design issues. Case management is a middle ground long-

term care policy reform option. Its implementation does not require fundamental changes in funding patterns or interorganizational relationships. The middle ground in which case management can be developed as a reform option is wider than present operational experience suggests. Models that expand case management to include authority for resource allocation and implementation of financial incentives to influence market conditions deserve greater attention.

We will look more closely at one type of discretion over resource control when we consider devolved budgets (below).

Johnson & Rubin (1983) consider that case management is particularly suited to meeting the needs of mentally ill people, especially those with long term needs which require regular monitoring. In Franklin et al (1987) a randomized pretest-posttest control group design was used to assign 417 individuals who had at least two discharges from a mental hospital to an experimental (E) group (N = 213) to receive case management services and a control (C) group (N = 204) who could receive any services but case management. After participation in the project for 12 months, 138 members of the E group and 126 members of the C group were reinterviewed. The E group received more services, cost more to maintain, and were admitted to mental hospitals more often, but concomitant improvement in quality of life indicators was not evident.

Dickey et al (1986) made a comprehensive cost comparison of resource utilization by seriously disabled chronic psychiatric patients randomly assigned to inpatient care and to an experimental residential program that provided an intermediate level of 24-hour care. At the end of the two-year study period, no significant changes in patients' clinical condition were observed, but costs for the experimental group averaged about $14,500 less (in 1981 dollars) than for the controls. The cost model included all treatment costs and nontreatment costs such as medical care, community services, case management, law enforcement and fire safety, maintenance outside the mental health system, and collateral costs.

The essential characteristics of the approach used by the Kent scheme in the UK (Davies & Challis, 1986) are:

co-ordination - between agencies
- of components of care/support
- of tasks (otherwise done by several people)

case-finding - offering service and removing impediments to those who should be recipients

screening - ensuring that referrals and recipients are in need and best helped by the service

assessment - multidisciplinary

care planning - and the arrangement of services and supports

monitoring - and if necessary adapting plans

gap identification - and filling by mobilising community resources or generating new, or altering old serv
ices.

A skilled case manager is able to see the early signs of deterioration in the client's circumstances and provide a stable relationship which is so often lacking in current service provision.
Case management relies on more than one mode of helping,
combines practical and therapeutic forms of help, makes use of
resources outside the statutory sector, and extends the responsibility for the costs of the service. This produces a quite different
set of incentives for professional workers, particularly social
workers. Of all the professionals at work in the community, social
workers probably exhibit more of the skills necessary to undertake this role. The coordinating role which they often play is
crucial to effective case management (Challis & Davies, 1986),
they have access to local authority resources, and are sometimes
adept at practical activity. The areas in which they would require
to develop the quality of their skills is in assessment, formulation
and care planning, review and monitoring.

The essence of the problem we face in the provision of welfare
services is an increasing diversity and loss of control, and so we
need a care system which enables better (more visible and more
effective) co-ordination to take place. Services which are required
to be cost-effective demand a system which increases awareness
of costs and enables flexibility in putting together packages of
care, tailoring these to the individual's needs. The PSSRU approach drew heavily on case management experiments in the
USA (in particular the Channelling initiative and similar
projects).

The PSSRU approach uses important devices to improve both
the effectiveness and the efficiency of case management. Devices
used in the scheme to improve the effectiveness of case management included: budgetary control (shadow pricing); the freedom
for social workers to introduce new or modify existing procedures; peer group support - to help social workers to consider the
separate elements of the approach (the recording system was
designed to help with this too); risk taking (which was more
acceptable and more expensive the greater the worker's experience); a manageable caseload; a recording system to reflect problem orientation, care planning and costs of items of care.

Devices which were used to improve the efficiency of the scheme (case management itself does not automatically lead to greater efficiency) were: shadow prices to improve workers understanding of costs; all services were nominally charged against the budget - to help to develop the ability to trade off the likely costs and benefits of different courses of action (gains in efficiency would help them to do more for those most in need); an unambiguous responsibility for each of the cases (this increases the visibility between agencies); and feedback of the information from the recording system (in peer groups) which increases the visibility of the work to the workers.

As in work with elderly people, the efficiency of a community mental health service is only likely to be improved if the service is regularly reviewed and properly coordinated. We have seen that all the major studies of after-care in the community mental health field show a similar picture of poor performance. The Homepack computer assisted coordination system developed in Hackney aims to improve the coordination of care services. We are involved with Derby Health Authority in an evaluation of the impact of the introduction of 'Homepack' into part of the Derby district. The levels of knowledge about services, and the involvement of different agencies is being assessed in two areas, and then Homepack is being introduced into one of them, and its impact assessed after several months in operation.

Problems with case management

Bachrach (1983) has warned of the dangers of assuming that case management can be used to provide a 'quick fix' for the problems of mental health care in the community. She points out that the role of the case manager can be separated from the concept of a case management system, and that in her view 'service integration' is a systems oriented concept to do with the interrelationships between programmes and agencies, whereas case management is a patient oriented concept. I think that she is really talking here about two different levels of 'system', the micro (patient) and the mezzo (agency). Her anxieties that natural caregiving networks might be supplanted by over-vigorous application of case management, and that it might introduce an unnecessary level of bureaucracy, do not seem to be borne out by the Kent findings.

Perhaps more problematic, in a mixed system of funding, is the means of ensuring that services which cross traditional boundaries remain accountable. Another issue, is the extent to which experimental programmes of case management can be translated into standard service provision. It is also clear form the experience of one of the post-Kent schemes that the essentials of case management and the type of skills necessary in order to carry it out are not really understood by some professionals. Case manager status was given to staff who, because of their training background and narrow focus of work, could not possibly comprehend the range of service possibilities, and who did not command the range of skills necessary to carry out assessment and care planning. The suggestion that GPs can carry out case management functions reveals the degree of misunderstanding about the breadth of the role of the case manager. The ability to perceive the gaps in service, and creative solutions, requires skill and influence of quite a different order.

How to ensure quality?

We did not introduce 'quality' as one of the elements in our model. Our main reason for not doing so was because we found it an elusive concept, which has connotations of 'excellence' or 'luxury' which are unhelpful. However, through the development of the concept of 'quality of life' and the notion of quality as 'conformance to requirements', (Crosby,1979) we think that there is some hope that quality may be studied more systematically.

Ultimately there must be an external arbiter of service quality. Internal arbiters are necessary, but are not sufficient. Private (for and not-for profit) agencies can be regulated. Where they are not regulated, market forces determine quality of care and agency survival. In the USA many states have deregulated the hospital building program, leading to an explosion in private psychiatric hospital care - 35% at the last count (cf. less than 10%) in 1970- in Utah, for example, as soon as deregulation took place, work began on eight new hospitals (Dorwart & Chartock,1988).

As Davies and Challis say, 'we have yet to learn the degree to which measures which would successfully achieve procedural accountability would produce a service of predictably high standard'. Many of the US case management projects included targeting criteria and eligibility; cost policies; approval of plans by clients and carers; training case managers etc. Some supported these procedures by independent reviews, and some of these reviews involved visiting samples of clients. The Channelling projects involved the following mechanisms:

Continued stay review (review of the appropriateness of continuing care and the determination of the correct level of that care)

Concurrent quality assurance (periodic review during which the care received by the patient is compared against criteria for performance developed by the professional community)

Medical care evaluation studies (retrospective audits of groups to compare the quality of care delivered against criteria of performance).

There are already some similar (perhaps less systematic) statutory and non-statutory developments like this in the UK - the role now played by the Social Services Inspectorate (SSI), the recommendations of Avebury's 'Home Life' document, the inspection and regulation of private homes by local authorities, and PASS.

Another approach is to attempt to create a standard based on the common conception of the diswelfares associated with various clinical conditions. This standard can then be used to compare the costs of different treatments. The Nottingham Health Index is one such scale, and the QALY is another. One year of healthy life counts as one qualy. The relative utility of various illness conditions in the Rosser/Kind index were made by 70 respondents, and were based on 8 states of disability and four levels of distress (Kind et al, 1982). Hurst (1988) has pointed out that the problems for this kind of analysis in the mental health field are: can mental illnesses be described unambiguously, and valued satisfactorily. The unreliability of diagnosis, and the failure of diagnosis to predict outcomes and service use suggest that other measures, of the disability associated with mental illnesses, or the social dysfunctions and diswelfares which accompany them might be better candidates for use in cost comparisons where improvements in health or welfare are the objective. One way of assessing these social factors is through the use of 'quality of life' measurement.

The idea that quality might be defined as 'conformance to requirements' begs such questions as 'whose requirements?' In the 'care sector' this cannot always be left to the consumer /customer alone. In some closely circumscribed circumstances clients do not always 'know what is best'. They may be unable to distinguish between alternative courses of action, both of which appear to be in the interests of his/her welfare, or their welfare may be at odds with what is in the best interests of someone else, perhaps in the same family. In most circumstances, however, the users requirements should be specified, and means must be devised to enable providers and purchasers of services to take account of their views in a systematic way.

Resource allocation and mental health services

The Reagan/Thatcher era has seen a preoccupation with cost containment (Ashbaugh,1981; Reamer, 1983), without a comparable interest in assuaging the enormous total cost of mental illness to all societies by providing better and more adequately resourced forms of care. Frank & Kamlet (1985) estimated that the total cost of mental illness care in the USA in 1980, was $50 billion dollars. The evidence that appropriate and timely psychiatric care reduces the cost of subsequent medical care seems to be ignored. Mumford et al (1984) have shown in their analysis of 23 existing studies that psychiatric care does reduce subsequent medical care costs, but mostly for those people who receive inpatient care and are over 55.

Reamer (1983) points out that in this essentially conservative era, shifting responsibility for care to the private sector is unlikely to make care for those who are difficult to help, or least likely to respond to treatment, any better or more available. There is growing evidence that the systems of financing health care in the USA, such as private insurance schemes and Health Maintenance Organisations (HMOs) lead to poorer services for mentally ill people.

Levin & Glasser (1984) in a survey of pre-paid mental health services found that 6% offered no mental health benefits, the variation in benefit was very great, and half did not have a person who was identified as responsible for mental health services. Sharfstein et al (1984) found that as fewer and fewer people could afford private psychiatric help, psychiatrists began to use 'less optimal treatment modalities' and to charge lower fees. Brady et al (1986) suggests that although more people are now covered by private insurance schemes, their benefits are tightly constricted. Hustead et al (1985) identified the scale of the reduction in benefit for mental and nervous illnesses. For instance in 1980, Blue Shield provided nearly full cover for in-patient care, but by 1983 this was limited to 60 days. Cheifetz & Salloway (1984) found the benefits provided by HMOs to be minimal, especially for out-patient care. Manning et al (1987) compared the use of out-patient services over time in an HMO and a fee-for-service plan. HMOs are believed to discourage psychiatric care seeking. A pre-paid system rather than a fee-for service system entirely alters the incentives associated with providing care, as Taube and Burns (1987) point out. Previously, under the fee for service system the more items of service on provided for the patient the more one was reimbursed and the more profit there was for the hospital. In the prospective payment system the more that is done for the patient the less the profit to the hospital.

A key feature in the Medicare system to reimburse hospitals for the care of elderly people is that the prospective payments are based on the resources allocated to care for different diagnostic groups (Diagnosis related groups (DRG); English et al, 1986). Psychiatric DRGs are very poor predictors of resource utilisation (see efficiency chapter). Schumacher et al (1986) found that only 4% of the cost of care could be attributed to diagnosis. Manning et al found that, although the use of the fee-for-service system and the HMO was the same in any one year, over time the HMO patients actually used 50% more services.

Pressure to reduce costs may result in the deployment of less expensive service providers, which may be efficient if the more expert providers' services were not really needed to achieve the same outcome, but which would be damaging if the cheaper provider did not achieve a comparable outcome for the client (Tulkin, 1982). Maynard (1989) (see below) sees some scope for this kind of substitution in primary care in the UK.

Rinella (1986) raises ethical questions in connection with cost containment strategies. Mental health services are often forced to employ less clinically qualified helpers in order to cut costs. Some treatment procedures are withdrawn, and the issue of 'effective' treatment is, he says, 'rarely raised'. In many cases less intensive treatment methods have been developed and, in some cases treatment options are chosen by administrators.

The various deficiencies of existing resource allocation methods leads some US authors to consider the possible advantages of a system of capitation payments (Lehman 1987) and voucher schemes (Talbott & Sharfstein, 1986). A useful discussion of the funding issue in a British context, in relation to the care of elderly people is given in Davies and Challis (1986; pp540-541).

Devolved budgets

In a commentary on the NHS White Paper in the UK (CM555, 1989) Maynard (1989) welcomes the clearer identification of the responsibilities of budget holders (hospital managers and GPs), and the long needed attempt to make managers and clinicians more cost conscious. He points out that currently cost differences are difficult to understand because of poor management information systems, but he thinks that there is cope for more efficiency in primary care, through generic prescribing; the substitution of cheaper labour; and an increase in list sizes.

Maynard also thinks that there will be a greater incentive to maximise the production of health (measured in terms of enhancement of duration and quality of life) at least cost, but worries that patient choice may be reduced because decisions about care options will be made by budget holders.

Accompanying the growth in the range of resource allocation systems is the tendency for smaller and more local sites of service provision to hold their own budgets. The size and scope of these budgets varies, but holding them has interesting social and psychological implications for the way in which services are provided. In many cases the budget holders are not trained in budget management, unless they have studied business or health administration. Clavner & Clavner (1987) regard this as the most glaring deficiency in the current US social work curriculum.

Professional staff may not have any more influence over a devolved budget than they did in the past, because they do not determine the size of the budget, merely its distribution. The psychological consequences, however, seem to be marked. Giving professional staff control of any part of their budget, however small, seems to have positive rather than negative consequences for professional practice, and, if the conclusions of studies in the field of service provision for the elderly are transferable to the mental health field, a positive benefit to clients and carers as well (Challis & Davies, 1986).

Having seen the Kent community care teams in operation and been an advisor to a subsequent PSSRU project, I can say that the acquisition of a devolved budget has been the single most influential factor in the improvement of practice that I have seen since I began to practice twenty years ago. There is no space here to go into the reasons for this in detail, but one self-evident feature of work with a devolved budget (however small and inadequate) is that it has a major effect on a person's feelings about 'locus of control'. It diminishes the worker's tendency to see other people, or an anonymous bureaucracy, as the only real source of shortage of resources and obstacles to success. Putting budgetary control back into the hands of clients presumably has something of a similar effect; it can be an enabling and an empowering development. Devolved budgetary control and a case management system can enable service providers and their clients to identify gaps in provision and shortfalls in welfare services, and make arguments for additional resources more purposeful as well as targeted at the specific gaps, rather than simply a never-ending plea for more resources.

Challis & Davies (1986) also note that the benefits of the devolved budget approach parallel the presumed benefits of geographical decentralisation. Unlike geographical decentralisation, which tends to handicap specialist work by making relations with agencies caring for groups of clients who have long term needs (who may be small in number in a geographical patch) more difficult, devolved budgets and case management actually improve contacts and relations between agencies.

Problems with devolved budgets

Having to distribute and account for a budget could conceivably draw attention away from the absolute size of the budget which is devolved. Williams & Williams (1987) point out that one disadvantage of implementing central control of devolved budget centres is that the budget holders become preoccupied with meeting financial targets at the expense of creative initiatives fundamental to long term objectives.

The question of who influences the spending of the budget

has been raised by Maynard (1989), and Hudson & Dubey (1986) argue that when central control assumes more importance community groups are left with less influence.

Conclusions

The main findings from the literature reviewed in this report lead us to draw the following conclusions. We make certain recommendations designed to avoid repeating the mistakes made in the USA.

We have seen that the meaning of 'CMHC' in the USA was a network of services, not a physical building, and we would advocate a similar usage in the UK, perhaps encouraging the use of the term 'community mental health services'. This term would encompass those provisions which are made by psychiatrists in hospital and community settings, and is wide enough to cover the contribution of the personal social services, the voluntary and private sectors, as well as user groups.

We have seen that the literature can be divided up into several reasonably discrete areas which correspond to major service principles and objectives. Principles and objectives may be shared by the various contributors to the community mental health service, and while they should be formally elaborated from time to time, they do not prescribe single solutions but may be achieved by a variety of types and combinations of forms of care.

The specification of minimum service coverage should be mandated, and joint proposals from social services, health, voluntary services and others should be approved in accordance with published standards. Community mental health services should be required to demonstrate that projects are genuinely collaborative before funds are released, and no service should be established without the means to provide adequate monitoring information and outside evaluation. The need for outside evaluation and the nature and broad content of monitoring should be mandated.

The quality of information relating to mental health service utilisation needs to be improved, and should be especially tailored to client need in this field not in general medicine. A more suitable system than the present one should be developed for mental health services, and research into a flexible, user-friendly, comprehensive mental health data-base is long overdue. This could combine the best of the old case-registers with modern PC technology, and co-ordinate what are currently rather piecemeal developments. A sophisticated modern system should be able to combine patient data with cost data, and relate both to small area statistics based on census and other local authority statistical information. In the absence of any better system of resource allocation, resources should be weighted towards areas of greatest social need. A valuable development would be a service information system which could combine clinical and non clinical information in a way which satisfies both the need for confidentiality and the requirements for data-protection.

The proportion of mental health expenditure allocated to acute sector psychiatric services should be reduced. This should be done by improving the level of expenditure on non-hospital services, and not only by transfer of funds from hospital closures which fosters the artificial division between hospital and community care.

Because community mental health services will be provided from a variety of sources, this network of services must have clear lines of accountability. Clients and carers should know the responsible person, and should have mechanisms to obtain redress if the system fails. One way of obtaining a clear understanding of the responsible party is to institute a case management system. The need for clear accountability exists just as much at the top, where there is a need for a minister responsible for health and 'human services'.

Serious consideration needs to be given to attempts to better co-ordinate services. Controlled experiments in the use of case management and other systems are necessary. Better means of assessing the true costs of these services are needed, and further work on appropriate and standardised methods of assessing the benefits of care are also required. Different systems of resource allocation should be systematically tested so that their implications for effective care in the community can be understood.

References

Ashbaugh, J.W. (1981) The Containment of Mental Health Centre Costs. *Administration in Mental Health* 9(1):46-56.

Austin, C. D. & Greenberg, Jay N. (1984) Comparing Case Management Systems. *Paper presented at the Annual Meeting of the Western Gerontological Society* (Anaheim, CA. March 17-21).

Austin, C. D. (1981) Case Management: Let Us Count the Ways. *Paper presented at the Joint Annual Meeting of the Scientific Gerontological Society* and the Scientific & Educational Canadian Association on Gerontology, Toronto, Ontario, Canada, November 8-12.

Bachrach, L.L. (1983) New Directions in deinstitutionalisation planning, In Bachrach, L.L. (ed) *Deinstitutionalisation* Jossey Bass, San Francisco.

Baier, M. (1987) Case management with the chronically mentally ill. *J Psychosoc Nurs Ment Health Serv* 25(6):17-20.

Brady, J., Sharfstein, S.S. & Muszynski, I.L. (1986) Trends in private insurance coverage for mental illness. *Am. J. Psychiat.* 143:1276-1278.

Challis, D. & Davies, B. (1986) *Case Management in Community Care* Gower, Aldershot.

Cheifetz, D.I. & Salloway, J.C. (1984) Patterns of mental health services provided by HMOs. *Am.Psychol.* 39:495-502.

Clavner, J.B. & Clavner, C. (1987) Motivating the Potential Social Worker. *Paper presented at the meeting of the Ohio College Association of Social Work Educators*, October 17.

CM555 (1989) *Working for Patients*, London, HMSO.

Crosby, P. (1979) *Quality is Free*. New York, McGraw-Hill.

Davies, B. & Challis, D. (1986) *Matching resources to needs in community care*. Aldershot, Gower.

Dickey, B., Cannon, N.L., McGuire, T.G., & Gudeman, J.E. (1986) The Quarterway House: a two-year cost study of an experimental residential program. *Hosp Community Psychiatry* 37 (11):1136-1143.

Dorwart,R.A. & Schlesinger,M. (1988) Privatization of psychiatric services. *Am.J.Psychiat.* 145(5):543-553.

English, J.T., Sharfstein, S.S., Scherl, D.J., Astrachan, B. & Muszynski, J.L. (1986) Diagnosis-related groups and general hospital psychiatry: The APA study. *Am.J.Psychiat.* 143:131-139.

Frank, R.G. & Kamlet, M.S. (1985) Direct costs and expenditures for mental health care in the US in 1980. *Hosp. Comm. Psychiat.* 36:165-168.

Franklin, J.L, Solovitz, B., Mason, M., Clemons, J.R. & Miller,G.E. (1987) An evaluation of case management. *Am J Public Health* 77 (6):674-678.

GAO (1988) Welfare Reform. Bibliographies of Case Management and Agency/Client Contracting. Fact Sheet for the Chairman, Committee on Governmental Affairs, U.S. Senate. *General Accounting Office*, Div. of Human Resources, Washington, D.C.

Garrison, C. (1986) Automated Performance Tracking and Productivity Improvement Project. Innovations in Protective Services. *Final Report*. Texas State Dept. of Human Resources, Austin.

Harris, M. & Bergman, H.C. (1987) Case management with the chronically mentally ill: a clinical perspective. *Am. J. Orthopsychiatry* 57(2):296-302.

Hudson, C.G. & Dubey, S.N. (1986) Decision Making under the ADAMHA Block Grant: Four case studies. *Administration Mental Health* 14:97-116.

Hurst, J. (1988) Economic Dimensions of Mental Health Evaluation In Marks et al (eds) *New Directions in Mental Health Care*. Institute of Psychiatry, London.

Hustead, E., Sharfstein, S., Muszynski, S., Brady, J. & Cahill,J. (1985) Reductions in coverage for mental and nervous illness in the Federal Employees Health Benefit Program 1980-1984. *Am.J.Psychiat.* 142:181-186.

Intagliata, J. & Baker, F.(1983) Factors Affecting Case Management Services for the Chronically Mentally Ill. *Administration in Mental Health* 11(2):75-91.

Johnson, P.J. & Rubin, A. (1983) Case Management in Mental Health: a social work domain? *Social Work* 281:49-56.

Kind, P., Rosser, R. & Williams, A. (1982) Valuation of Quality of Life: Some Psychometric Evidence. In Jones-Lee, M.W. (ed) *The Value of Life and Safety*.

Lehman, A.F. (1987) Capitation payments and mental health care: a review of the opportunities and risks. *Hosp.Comm. Psychiat.* 38:31-38.

Levin, B.L. & Glasser, J.H. (1984) A national survey of pre-paid mental health services. *Hosp.Comm.Psychiat.* 35:350-355.

Manning, W.G., Wells, K.B. & Benjamin, B. (1987) Use of outpatient mental health services over time in HMO and fee-for-service plans. *Am.J.Psychiat.* 144:283-287.

Marlowe, H. A., Jr. (1983) The Mental Health Counsellor as Case Manager: Implications for Working with the Chronically Mentally Ill. *American Mental Health Counsellors Association Journal* 5(4):184-191.

Maynard, A. (1989) Carrots to blend with choice cuts. *Guardian*, January 30, p16.

McDaniel, G. (1986) Case Decision Project. *Final Report* (Process Evaluation). Texas State Dept. of Human Resources, Austin.

Morris, J. (1987) Housing and case managed home care programs and subsequent institutional utilisation.*Gerontologist* 27(6):788-796.

Mumford, E., Schlesinger, H.J., Glass, G.V., Patrick, C. & Cuerdon, T. (1984) A new look at evidence about reduced cost of medical utilisation following mental health treatment. *Am.J.Psychiat.* 141:1145-1158.

Raschko, R. (1985) Systems Integration at the Program Level: Aging and Mental Health. *Gerontologist* 25(5):460-463.

Reamer, F.G. (1983) Social Services in a Conservative Era. *Social Casework* 64:451-458.

Rinella, V. (1986) Ethical issues and psychiatric cost containment strategies. *Int.J. Law Psychiatry* 9:125-136.

Schumacher, D.N., Namerow, M.J., Parker, B., Fox, P. & Kofie, V. (1986) Prospective payment for psychiatry: feasibility and impact. *New England Journal of Medicine* 315:1331-1336.

Seltzer, M. M. (1987) Family Members as Case Managers: Partnership Between the Formal and Informal Support Networks. *Gerontologist* 27(6):722-728.

Sharfstein, S.S., Eist, H., Sack, L. Kaiser, H. & Shadoan, R.A. (1984) The impact of third party payment cutbacks on the private practice of psychiatry: Three surveys *Hosp.Comm.Psychiat.* 35:478-481.

Talbott, J.A. & Sharfstein, S.S. (1986) A proposal for future funding of chronic & episodic mental illness. *Hosp. Comm. Psychiat.* 37:1126-1130.

Taube, C.A. & Burns, B.J. (1988) Cross-national evaluations of mental health services delivery and financing: some collaboration opportunities. In Marks et al (eds) *New Directions in Mental Health Care.* Institute of Psychiatry, London.

Tulkin, S.R. (1982) Therapists' contributions to program development in an HMO. *Paper presented to the Annual Convention of the American Psychological Association* (Washington, DC, August, 23-27.

Wagner, W.G. (1987) Child Sexual Abuse: A Multidisciplinary Approach to Case Management. *Journal of Counselling & Development* 65(8):435-439.

Williams, K. & Williams, J. (1987) M-Way crash. *Times Higher Ed.Suppl.* October 16.

Wilson, N. L. (1983) Serving Impaired Elders in the Community: The Interface of Case Management with Mental Health Services. Texas Project for Elders: Assistance with Long Term Care. *Paper presented at the Annual Scientific Meeting of the Gerontological Society* (San Francisco, CA. November 17-22).

Wright, R.G., Sklebar, H.T, & Heiman, J.R. (1987) Patterns of case management activity in an intensive community support program: the first year. *Community Mental Health Journal* 23 (1):53-59.

Index

Dightman, 190
Dinitz, 148
Dinkel, 66, 71, 167, 170 - 172
Disability, 88, 108, 136, 203
Discrimination, 21
Disgnostic, 96
Dittmar, 145
Donovan, 25, 44
Dorwart, 56, 202, 209
Doty, 175, 194
Dowds, 125, 145
Dowell, 13, 17, 18, 20, 38, 41, 44, 53, 56, 57, 61, 65, 69, 72, 76, 113, 121, 122, 141, 145, 152, 153, 172
DRG, 95, 113, 117, 204
Driggers, 193
Drop-in, 162
Drude, 30, 48, 181, 183, 184, 194
DSM-III, 116, 146
Dubey, 207, 210
Dumpman, 193
Durlak, 165, 172
Dush, 185, 190
Dutch, 5, 27, 114
Dyck, 125, 145

Edwards, 93
Effective services, 2, 3, 7 - 9, 11, 14, 26 - 28, 33, 34, 49, 52, 63, 71, 79, 89, 90, 91, 93, 110, 111, 122, 123, 127, 132, 140, 141, 147, 150, 157, 164, 165, 179, 182, 197, 200, 205, 208
Effectivenes, 182
Effectiveness, 3, 14, 20, 22, 23, 28, 31, 32, 36, 41, 44, 76 - 80, 83, 89, 94, 99, 111, 115, 119 - 125, 129, 131, 134, 140 - 143, 147, 150, 152 - 155, 165, 172, 174, 178, 180, 182, 185, 188, 200
Efficiency, 9, 14, 17, 23, 25, 26, 28, 41, 54, 56, 76, 77, 79, 80, 84, 85, 89, 93 - 100, 103 - 105, 108, 110 - 123, 144, 153 - 156, 174, 180, 183, 200, 201, 204, 205
Eist, 211

Elderly people, 6, 18, 29, 31, 32, 34, 35, 39, 57, 94, 132, 134, 197, 198, 201, 204 - 206
Elkins, 28, 48
Ellis, 180, 190
Ellsworth, 185, 190
Emergency services, 5, 11, 15, 18, 19, 28, 31, 41, 45, 51, 60, 61, 62, 72, 75, 81, 83, 84, 90, 101, 141
Employment, 17, 20, 88, 102, 108, 127, 165, 170
Empowerment, 160
Endicott, 146, 175
Epidemiology, 112, 114 - 117
Equality, 75, 153
Erbinger, 44
Erdman, 100, 113
Essex, 159, 170, 172
Ethnic minorities, 8, 11, 47, 52, 53, 55, 56, 64 - 66, 69, 72, 97, 98, 126, 160
Etzioni, 177, 191
Evaluation, 1 - 5, 10 - 12, 16, 22, 26, 30, 31, 43 - 48, 71 - 75, 78, 83, 92, 112 - 119, 121, 123, 133, 137, 142, 144 - 150, 154, 159, 160, 166 - 181, 184 - 196, 201, 202, 207, 209, 210
Evans, 114, 117
Eysenck, 19, 44

Fagin, 179, 191
Fairbank, 95, 115
Fairweather, 127, 145
Fakhouri, 82, 115
Falloon, 122, 132, 145
Faragher, 114
Farber, 60, 72
Farndale, 46
Featheringham, 187, 193
Feldman, 4, 5, 6, 11, 13, 16, 20, 24, 33, 40, 41, 44, 178, 191
Feldstein, 85, 113
Fenton, 21, 89, 113
Ferlie, 58
Fernandez, 176, 191
Fernando, 162
Fiester, 4, 11, 35, 45, 61, 72

223